WHY YOU SHOULD READ TH

1. You won't find anything else like it: and videos that depict med student life ~~g~~ ~~source~~ out there that gives an in-depth account of the first year medical school experience.

2. The first year of medical school is a survival of the fittest: Even after months of proving to ad coms why you're qualified enough to be accepted, the learning curves for information and life lessons are STEEP. From your first day forward, you will be thrust into a world of barely-sensible acronyms and strange lingo; and it's pretty much left up to chance for you to somehow adjust to this cut-throat career while maintaining your grades, your personal life, and your sanity. This process can be very unforgiving and distressing, especially without the right resources and support to keep you in the fight.

3. The first year of med school is the most critical year of a physician's career: This is when study/learning habits are formed, the foundations of professionalism and teamwork are established, and when you decide if you're down for the long haul of board exams, bureaucracy, constant evaluations, endless hours of learning and training, and another application season at the end of med school.

4. Practicing physicians who give med students advice (and rightfully so) forget the juicy details of what their first year was like. No shade: Most of the "I-wish-I-had-done's" are lost in the whirlwind of just barely surviving their first year, boards, and clerkships, leaving out the key details of some important lessons and tips. The advice from a first-year med student couldn't be fresher.

5. Med school does NOT happen in a vacuum: Many believe that there is no room for personality, advocacy, service, or acknowledgments of disparities and injustice in med school, let alone during the first year. WRONG. First year is a critical turning point in learning how to infuse your passions and perspectives into your career.

6. Simply "pushing harder" does not guarantee success in medical school. It only guarantees burnout: The world needs more whole physicians who haven't been dragged and drained through med school for four straight years in a row. A collective move toward pass/fail standardized tests and curricula is sufficient proof that a holistic and authentic approach to being successful in medical school is a healthier alternative to the traditional methods.

7. Good medical education resources don't have to be so stuffy, so imma keep it real and make it plain.

Doctah-ing it Up.

A Guide for Adapting to the Culture of Medicine in Your First Year of Medical School

JA'NEIL G. HUMPHREY

Author's Disclaimer:

All my opinions are my own. I do not claim to have all of the answers. All advice, suggestions, and tips are derived from my own experiences. Some topics were inspired by conversations shared with family members, therapists, and counselors. This information is not intended to replace counsel from therapists, advisors, educators, or clergy.

I acknowledge that everyone's path is different and unique and do not claim that all methods and suggestions apply to all medical students. Although this guide is for students of all cultural backgrounds, I intend that this guide will normalize the shared obstacles of the medical school experience for black, first-generation medical students like me; and will highlight aspects of the BIPOC experience in medical education. In doing so, I hope to encourage and inspire the next generation of dope physicians.

ISBN: 978-0-578-99446-8

Cover Design: Jasmine Haddad

Published in the United States of America

To the first-generation med students who are breaking the mold to build a family legacy.

To my brothas and sistas in medicine just tryna raise that 5%.

To my village. I am because you are.

And to my mother—my "ming", my momager, my prayin' mama, and reason behind the title of the book."Thank you" will never be enough.

contents

section 1

section 2

section 3

The Art of Doctah-ing it Up: 53
Growing into the Role of "Doctor"

section 4

Creating a Balanced Med Student Lifestyle   71

section 5

section 6

section 7

appendix

Contributors & Editors

A special thanks to these awesome folk who helped make this guide possible:

Jasmine Haddad, medical student— cover art

Shantal Tummings, medical student

Sierra Garrett, medical student

Joseph Smittick, medical student

Aurriel Fenison, medical student

Ashley Saunders, medical student

Isabelle Kaneza, medical student

Yamiko J. Chanza, medical student

Clifton Jessup Jr.

Tino Mkorombindo, MBA

Pamela O'Garro-Humphrey, MSW

Timothy Young, MD

Deena Bengiamin, MD

Amy Hayton, MD, MPH

Jessica ChenFeng, PhD, LMFT

Welcome

My name is Ja'Neil ("juh-NEEL") and I'm sending you love and light from Southern California where I'm a second-year med student.

Before we get right into it, let me tell you about myself: I'm a proud second-generation Caribbean gyal from Jersey, Christian, HBCU alumna, oldest of two, and plant mom of nineteen (and counting).

As a kid, ya girl was *artsy artsy*, and everyone was convinced that I would be a singer, dancer, model, or something along those lines. I mean who could blame them? I was a pageant girl who sang at every kind of venue you could think of and was classically trained in ballet and jazz dance. The works. Even I was convinced that my path to a career on the stage was a sure thing. Next thing you know, God said "I see what you're tryna do....but you're gonna be a doctor."

Plot twist.

And so, I fell in love with science in my junior year of high school and I declared that I was going to be a surgeon. Just like that. I didn't even know what it would take or how long I would have to be in school. You're talking about a girl who didn't have any doctors in her family (except for a very distant aunt), pretty much lived at the dance studio, and had ZERO knowledge about science; yet I dedicated the next fifteen years of my life to medicine before I could even drive.

Call it foresight, divine inspiration, or even insanity, but when my mind was made up, there was no turning back. And ever since, I've never been able to see myself being anything other than a physician. At first, this was quite the undertaking because I declared a demanding career that I didn't know jack about. So initially, I went through all the confusion that came with figuring out what the heck an "MCAT" was, why I had to do this boring thing called research, and why there were so many acronyms for everything in science. Compared to my art background—characterized by expressionism, chord progressions, and *en dedans* pirouettes—medicine was a whole new world. And *lawd*, there were so many times when I doubted that I was on the right path.

However, I always knew deep down that there were other people just like me with the same dream and no idea how to make it happen. Secondly, I took one look at the percentage of practicing black physicians and the admission and dropout rates for black students in medical school, realized that this path was less traveled than I thought, and concluded that I had to stay in the fight to change this. Lastly, I knew that learning what it *really* meant to do this doctor thing with no frame of reference could put others, who might be just as shook as I was, at an advantage. So, with all things considered, I started soaking up all of the knowledge and advice I could find to empower myself and others coming up behind me. The same girl who at one point didn't know an artery from a vein decided to apply to medical school and mentor high school and college students to do the same. Wild.

Fast forward to 2021 where I'm days into my second year of medical school at Loma Linda University in California. In addition to trying to survive second year, I currently co-lead a Longitudinal Pre-med Mentorship Program (LPMP) for my school's community, and serve as the Student National Medical Association (SNMA) Minority Association of Premedical Students (MAPS) Associate Regional Director for the mighty Region 1. I also serve on the executive board for Greater Influence, a student-led non-profit that offers MCAT prep materials, mentorship, workshops, and financial support for pre-medical students. Although it has been a wild ride and my story is far from over, I've been abundantly blessed thus far while making seats at the table for underrepresented and non-traditional students like me, as I make one for myself.

Even though I now know a little bit more about the medical school journey than I did in high school (or at least enough to write a book about it) my goals haven't changed that much. I still see my future self in the operating room changing the culture of medicine one cut at a time, and I see you there too— as an example that unique pathways to success shape the medical field to reflect the *real* world.

So, I hope that after reading these 100-sumthin' pages of advice, you will have the same amount of confidence in yourself that I have in you to apply nothing but pressure during these next four years of med school.

Congratulations!

Now, enough about me. Congratulations on getting accepted into medical school! If you didn't already know, this is high-key a big deal. Big ups to you.

Regardless of the school you were at before, what your MCAT score or GPA was, or how many gap years you took, you now have a clean slate. You have respawned, but this time, with your white coat.

Spoiler alert: If you're type-A like me, you came across this guide because you want to make sure you're 100% prepared for medical school. But here's the tea: that's not possible (okay maybe you can be 80% ready-ish). But what I *can* guarantee is that a smooth transition is in your reach if you remain true to yourself every step of the way.

How do you go about doing so?

That's where I come in. Think of me as your med school auntie-guide.

First, take a deep breath. You're gonna need it.

Now let's get started.

How To Get the Most Out of this Guide

- Take everything in it with a grain of salt.
- When applying the tips you learn, please do so gradually.
- When you start to feel overwhelmed, you've read too much.
- Take the tools from it and make them you're own.
- Pass on what you've learned to someone else.

Helpful Tools & Features

Major Keys: As much as it hurt me to put this tired DJ Khaled reference here, the bolded paragraphs in each section are major keys for first year.

THE BOTTOM LINE: This feature is at the end of each section and highlights the most important takeaways.

Additional Resources: I do not have all of the answers and can only share my perspective, so at the end of each section, I left you some additional books and things to help you if you need a deeper dive into what we cover.

First Year Checklist: This is the first thing you'll find in the appendix and is a cheat sheet to make sure you have everything you need to start medical school.

"Med-Speak" Glossary: This is the second item you'll find at the end of the guide. This has all of the lingo that is helpful for you to know in your first year— because if you don't already know, doctah speak is a whole 'nother language.

Hierarchy of Medicine: The third item at the end that outlines the *who's who* of medicine.

To start, here is a list of some things you're likely to encounter in your first (MS1/M1) year regardless of what medical school you attend:

- **The white coat ceremony:** This is where you receive your "short coat". Often thought of as a right of passage, this ceremony symbolizes the responsibility you now have as an icon of health and leadership. This is also the time to flex, so take as many pics as possible.

- **Anatomy lab:** The only place on earth where it's okay to get hungry while looking at dismembered body parts. This is where you will see your "first patient", who will have a higher pain tolerance than you'd expect.

- **Practical exams:** Depending on your curriculum and school-specific requirements, you'll be tested on the identification of histology (tissue) slides, EKGs, and more. These will be similar to the lab finals you had in undergrad—just ten times harder, of course.

- **OSCEs:** Pronounced "ah-skees", Objective Structured Clinical Examinations, are how you'll be evaluated against the national standards for physical exams and patient interviews. *See pg. 45*

- **Humbling test grades:** No one comes to medical school knowing everything. If they say or act like they do, trust me they're either lying or faking it. Everyone's first test is TRASH. Basura. But trust me, it will get better as you get comfortable troubleshooting your learning methods. (There's a whole section on that a little later on; see *section 2*.)

- **Diagnosing yourself:** You'll often question whether or not you have palpitations, a rare skin lesion you just learned about, the mental condition your lecture just covered, or all of them at the same time.

- **Imposter syndrome:** This condition is the one you *should* be worried about. It's going to take a minute before it hits you that you'll be somebody's doctor soon. And when it does, you may suddenly forget all the reasons why you deserve to be where you are. *See pg.61*

- **Sleep deprivation**: Always stay strapped with your coffee and Red Bull in hand.

- **Your "aha" moment:** One day it will all start to "click". You may not understand everything, but you'll eventually get used to the pace and volume of material. And man, that feeling is one of the best there is. Don't stop searching for that moment until it comes.

- **FOMO:** Short for "fear of missing out"; everyone's life outside of your med school bubble is going to look more exciting than yours while you're slaving over lectures and studying all weekend. Just remember, there will be nothing more rewarding than having someone calling you "doctor so-and-so" in a few years. Beloved, you are here for both a good time and a long time, so buckle in.

- **"The Devil's Seven Weapons":** A wise friend of mine once told me that starting every new chapter in life will come with its share of these seven things:
  - **Deception:** Not everyone will be who they say they are. Be smart about who and what you associate with. *Be as wise as a serpent and as harmless as a dove.*
  - **Distraction:** Staying focused is a constant battle. Know that you can win. Every. Single. Time.
  - **Doubt:** Some days you will doubt if you're meant to be where you are. Cling to people, thoughts, and values that destroy your doubt.
  - **Discouragement:** Your grades and scores may not always reflect your effort, but every day is a new day to succeed.
  - **Death:** You're likely at an age when so much is changing in your life. You may lose family members, friends, pets, and things that mean so much to you. But from here on out, there will never be a "right time" to

experience and cope with loss. During these seasons, find your circle and lean on them. More specifically, this career will have a weird way of acquainting you with the causes and results of death as you learn about the human body.

- **Distortion:** Your truth will be constantly challenged. Stay rooted.
- **Darkness:** I witnessed firsthand how easy it can be to find yourself in a place where the first six things come at you all at the same time. When you can't be the light, run toward it. Crawl if you have to. Always remain connected to what allowed you to get to this point. Frequently read your personal statement. Renew your faith in Christ. Give back through service. Do whatever you have to until a light is relit in you.

A GLIMPSE INTO SECOND YEAR

Everything you learn (study habits, centering techniques, testing stamina, and the information you'll be taught in class from day 1) should prepare you to take your United States Medical Licensing Exam (USMLE) Step 1 exam, which will most likely take place right after your second year of didactics (non-clinical years).

Thankfully, if you're reading this, Step 1 has already been changed to pass/fail which means that you DON'T, I repeat you DO NOT have to start studying in-depth for this exam until your dedicated period (a time specifically set aside to studying for boards) at the end of your second year. It also means that living a balanced life is a realistic goal and will set the tone for the next few years.

THE BOTTOM LINE

Although most MS1s experience similar milestones, success during first year (and your entire med school experience) is a reflection of your **balance, efficiency, focus,** *and* **self-awareness.** (Notice how I didn't say anything about grades and studying...yet).

I'd be lying if I said that following every single piece of advice I give you to a tee will make your first year a breeze. But maximizing the four areas I mentioned **in your unique way** will set an unshakable foundation for your success in med school. That's a promise that you can take straight to the bank.

section 1
A Different World:
Getting Orientated & Acclimated

Navigating A New Environment

At the beginning of my first year of medical school, moving from bipolar-weathered New Jersey to always-sunny Southern California was stressful. I was on my own in a new place and on a new coast for the first time. I hate to admit it, but even after three weeks of my mom helping me get situated in my new environment, I cried like a baby the whole way back from LAX the day she left.

COVID-19 also added to the struggle of getting settled in this new community because so many places were closed. Also, at that time, there was no vaccine available.

But what did I do anyway? I tried to recreate the lifestyle I had in undergrad, which I quickly found out did not work (Trust me, I have better common sense these days).

After twenty-two years, it was time to officially cut the cord.

I did everything I could to get a feel of the area before arriving: Googling how far Walmart was away from campus, reaching out to current students to see what neighborhoods I should look for apartments in, and seeing how close the beaches were, etc. But no matter how much I prepped, arriving early helped me construct a realistic idea of how my life would be in this new place.

Identifying a few key places before classes start will help you settle into a new city:

- 99 Cents stores
- Beauty supply
- Farmer's market
- African market
- Your pharmacy
- Cleaners
- Car wash
- Church
- Coffee shop
- Gym

Living Arrangements & Roommates

If you're used to being miles away from home or adapting to new environments, this section may not provide you with any new information. However, if you're anything like me—super type-A, stubborn, a never-lived-far-away-from-family kind of person, this section is just for you.

Comfort is key

When you're deciding if a place is a good housing option for you, ask yourself how much studying, peace, or productivity is possible there. If the answer is very little, consider how realistic it is to drive somewhere to put in long study hours whenever you need to.

What I'm about to say may be common sense, but you may need to hear this. Your place should be your escape and your safe space. It should fit your aesthetic and should feature an area that is just for you (for my island folk, *smallin' up ya self* should be the LAST resort). In other words, if you can't break down and cry and shout, have a moment of silence, or feel free to be yourself, you shouldn't live there.

I also realize that this may be the first time you're living on your own, and in a place that has your name on the lease at that. Here are a few things you should consider when looking for a place:

- Distance from your school/ traffic patterns
- Safety and overall vibes of the complex / neighborhood
- Promotional period windows (how much will rent increase next year?)
- Renter's insurance
- Additional rental expenses (water, rent, utilities, internet, TV, trash disposal, maintenance costs)

We'll talk about this again later in section 7, but each institution has a pre-determined amount that is available to you every year you apply for loans. If you can't receive rent assistance from your parents, this amount should be considered when finding an apartment within your budget.

A Word on Roommates

I have NEVER heard of a roommate situation that just "worked" without any form of communication or verbalized expectations. If you're clean and your roommate says they are too, nine times out of ten the word "clean" means two completely things to the both of you.

When moving in with a new roommate, draw up a contract or list of expectations and agree on it within the first week of move-in day. This may seem harsh, but it will save you so much frustration (that I have experienced in the past) that you do not need in your first year of medical school. Also, it will set the tone for effective communication between you and your roommate.

Even before agreeing to move in with them, meet with them for a cup of coffee at Starbucks or something to make sure they're not weird or "off". DO NOT wait until the lease is signed to get to know them, even if you've seen them once before or chatted with them over text. You'll thank yourself (and me) later on

for making sure your roommate is a person you can trust and feel comfortable around. You may have come across similar lists online or a roommate quizzes in undergrad, but here are a few topics that you should *actually* discuss with your potential roommate:

Fool-Proof Roommate Questions

- Are you more clean than neat or more neat than clean?

- How do you plan on upkeeping the common areas every week? Do you prefer leaving most housework until the end of the week?

- Do you pay bills on time or take full advantage of the grace period?

- Do you plan on hosting events or study sessions at the house? How often might those happen?

- What were your previous experiences with roommates like?

- Is there is a time or times during the day you prefer to be left alone?

- What are your non-negotiables?

- Do you have any allergies to food or pets?

- What is your living aesthetic?

- What is your understanding of what I will be doing in medical school? (not everyone understands what med school is like and what that will require of you)

On a serious note, don't just say that you're "flexible" because if you're not, you'll be miserable.

The easiest, less rigid way to find a roommate with similar values is to room with another medical student. It's an even better idea to seek out a third or fourth-year roommate for guidance and resources that may serve you well in your first year.

Whatever you do, cling to your standards and expectations when choosing someone to live with. I cannot stress this enough because you'll need every brain cell you can muster to pass your classes.

After all of my previous successful and unsuccessful roommate interactions, I decided to live alone during my first year. And chil', it was worth every nickel and dime of loan money.

Living Alone
If you decide to go solo like I did, make sure you get to know your neighbors, the leasing agent, the owner even, and the maintenance staff. You still need someone looking out for you, especially if you are a female living by yourself. Make sure that someone has a copy of your key. If there is no one you trust enough to

do that, mail a copy to your parents just in case or keep a spare key somewhere secret.

Renting a Room
Renting a room is a great option for first year. I rented one while I was still looking for an apartment, and I have many classmates who found that this arrangement worked for them for the entire year. Again, make sure expectations on household responsibilities and costs are worked out weeks before your move-in day. The last thing you want is to get trapped in an unideal situation without a lease agreement to fall back on.

Living at Home
From what I have heard, living at home during medical school is a FLEX. If I could, I would, even when considering the stigma that many of my classmates felt about living with their parents during the prime of their adult life.

I don't know about you, but there is nothing like having full access to home-cooked meals, FREEEE RENT, and a support system right there during low moments. But of course, it does come with its cons too.

One thing I've heard from classmates living at home is that setting healthy boundaries is the key to making living at home work. This entails not feeling bad when you aren't available to run errands or can't complete as many house chores as before.

Although I was miles away from my family, I also had to set boundaries with them to secure my success in first year. (*there's more on boundaries in section 5*)

The Med School Supplies You *Actually* Need

Depending on what your coins are looking like, you should invest in some med school must-haves:

- **Srubsssss:** You can splurge a little on WearFigs or you can go to your local thrift store. I did both. You'll definitely need this for labs or days when you don't feel like putting on actual clothes.

- **A lab coat:** It's good to have a long one that goes down to your knees for anatomy lab. Doesn't have to be anything too fancy. Having a coat you don't mind getting cadaver juices on is what you're going for. Your school may give you a used one for free, so make sure you ask around.

- **Stethoscope:** You DON'T need to buy a stethoscope unless your school requires you to. You'll probably be told to purchase a complete set of medical supplies from their standardized vendor of choice. If this is the case, all you'll need is a bag for all of your supplies.

- **A sturdy bag:** I invested in a tote bag that doubles as a backpack. Cool right? (*this is me trying to validate my decision to spend half a band on a bag for school*). But seriously, this is a must.

Whatever you decide to buy doesn't have to be as elaborate but should be just as durable and versatile. It will come in handy on those days that you have multiple appointments or classes on campus. If you're looking for a trendy alternative, a large canvas bag will work just fine.

- **Noise-canceling headphones/ ear-muffs/ earplugs:** Until you find a golden study spot, noise-canceling headphones will help you focus at the local coffee shop or library.

- **A planner:** An absolute essential. Phone calendars are cool, but physically writing boosts recall.

- **A good-quality tumblr:** Somehow your body uses up water ten times faster when you start medical school, so investing in a large Hydro Flask or water jug will help you stay hydrated throughout the day.

- **A watch:** For some reason, I refuse to get an Apple Watch until it's time for clinical rotations, but whatever floats your boat will work. My retro Casio watch beeps every hour to help me assess my study progress throughout the day. Plus it was only 20 bucks.

- **Power bank:** You'll thank me later.

- **Tablet/ Laptop:** It will be a challenge not having either of these, but having one or the other will work. If you're considering using a tablet as your primary device, investing in a good-quality keyboard is a good move.

- **Tablet stylus:** Again, if you'll be taking the majority of your notes on your tablet, it will be helpful to get a stylus that makes the writing experience as realistic as possible. Purchasing a paper-like screen protector for your tablet is also a good option.

- **Protection/holsters for your devices:** This was essential for me, considering my track record for unintentionally scratching and breaking screens. I purchased tons of laptop and phone screen protectors and new cases to make sure that in the frenzy of my new life as a med student, I wouldn't damage the devices I couldn't afford to replace. If you know this is also you, don't play ya self, and add them to your Amazon cart ASAP.

- **Extra pens and pencils:** You don't have to go all out like you did the first day of middle school but just make sure you're always prepared.

- **Dry-erase markers:** (and access to a whiteboard): Really important for studying on the go.

- **A versatile pair of dress shoes:** You should aim to strike a balance between comfort and style in every pair of shoes you wear because you never know what the long days on campus may bring. *(more on pg. 69)*

- **Cushions for your toosh:** You'll be studying at your desk for hours on end. Make sure your back and bum have enough support.

- **Blue light glasses:** Be kind to your eyes. They will thank you.

- **A box of masks:** Hopefully, by the time you start your first year, COVID-19 herd immunity will be achieved, but if not, keeping a stash or two of masks is a good idea. The same goes for hand sanitizer—get some for the house, the car, and for your bag.

Everything else you see your classmates and other med influencers buy (suture kits, pins, fancy pen lights, and reflex hammers, etc.) are usually bells and whistles to flex, that's all. So, don't worry if some of these items aren't in your budget.

Always check with your school for an official list of things you need to buy and or what will be provided to you.

whispers in broke med student the thrift store also has some great stuff, some of which is brand. Spaking.New.

THE BOTTOM LINE

If you're not completely comfortable in your new environment, first year will be very ghetto. A drag. Akin to pulling teeth.

Out of all the new things you will experience, knowing your way around your new environment, settling on a comfortable living situation, and having the necessary supplies will give you the sense of normalcy you need to stay grounded.

section 2
Beating the Learning Curve with Buckets

The Fire Hydrant

My least favorite phrase of first year was "MeDiCaL sCHooL is LikE DriNkinG oUt of a FiRe hyDrAnT" You'll probably hear this a lot too. So me, being as type-A as can be, was determined to defeat the odds by:

1. Placing a whole bunch of buckets out under the water so I could catch a lot of information at once

2. Rearranging and storing the buckets in a way that played to my strengths

3. Pouring all I could carry in the buckets out of them when it was time to do so

Yea. I know I took the bucket thing pretty far, but it worked. It was the framework I used to develop a system of organized chaos, triaging, and compartmentalization to academically adapt, which may work for you too.

I am happy to report that the information you will learn in medical school is NOT HARD. It is not some code to crack nor is this unattainable wealth of knowledge only accessed by the smartest of them all.

You will find that the real challenge in med school is the volume of information thrown at you all at once, rather than the difficulty of the information itself.

Remember, you made it to medical school because you can understand how science generally works, so you have more than enough to build on from day one.

Your goal shouldn't be to just know a lot of facts but to know *how* to learn those facts well.

This leads to another spoiler alert: YOU CAN'T MEMORIZE EVERYTHING! But, you can create mental frameworks that will help you retrieve as much information as possible. Hence the buckets.

Hate to break it to you, but if you thought you did all you could to study in undergrad, you're in for a big surprise. One thing about med school is that it will expose the problems in your study strategies that were masked by all the time you had in undergrad.

This means that what you did to learn in college will not work. Point blank period. Even after your study regimen changes in the first few weeks of medical school, it will change again and again as you adapt to stress and change itself.

When I first realized this, it hit me like a truck. It seemed impossible to "reinvent" my study approach over and over again. It was so annoying to constantly try new strategies because most of them didn't last a week before they were replaced.

My study approach was completely different for EVERY test cycle in my first year. But, it was worth it to find out what unique mixture of techniques worked for me. By the end of the year, these core methods were constants no matter what strategies I used:

1. Staying **ahead of lectures** from the start so I could use test week for REVIEW ONLY
2. Using strategies that maximize **active learning** (e.g. annotating lecture notes and asking myself questions about material DURING each lecture) to stay engaged and awake.
3. **Weekly summary sheets** with questions and correlations I made during the week
4. Summary **diagrams of major concepts** for physiology and pathophysiology. *See pg. 34*

There are more details on what this looked like later on in this section.

Overall, I included things in my routine that helped me overcome common obstacles to learning.

You should too, especially if you are at ground zero (after being humbled by a low first test grade, for example).

Collecting as Much Water as You Can: Overcoming Obstacles to Learning

As you begin to think about the most effective and efficient ways to learn concepts, first, think about what your greatest obstacles to learning are historically. Here are some common obstacles and some possible solutions to them:

Obstacle #1 | Too many details to memorize for one topic, a medical condition, or a drug:

The easy answer is to make a bunch of mnemonics. But sometimes everything about a topic won't fit into a catchy phrase.

Another option is to make a story about each condition or drug with wacky, out-of-the-box details that will help you remember the key points. These don't have to make sense to anyone except for you.

For example, to remember Paget's disease of bone, which is frequently found in people 50 years and older, I imagined a middle-aged French painter named Paget ("pah-JEH") who was "se-que-tly"—as in secretly—sick (to remember that SQST1 is mutated) *Cues montage*

Paget was a painter on the run. He refused to get vaccinated because he thought that being sick would ruin his fame. But, no matter how hard he tried, the **weasels** and **whistleblowers** of each town he moved to somehow found out that he was sick (it can be caused by a bone infection with Measles and can cause hearing loss).

Every time this happened, he ran away **faster than** the townspeople could confront him about his secret (in this disease, bone remodeling occurs at a faster rate than bone formation resulting in weaker bones).

And to make matters worse, all of the streets in France were **cement** (cement lines are a characteristic feature) and so every time he ran his **bones and heart** became weaker (high output cardiac failure is a common feature of Paget's).

If this seems like a lot, there are great resources (that I'll mention a bit later) that already have premade, illustrated, and animated stories like this one to help you remember different conditions and drugs.

It may not be efficient to make a story for everything you learn in first year, but until you get better at learning the patterns of pathogenesis (*how* things go wrong) and pathways, this method may work in the meantime.

Obstacle #2 | Difficulty understanding all of the big words and "medical talk":

Seek out multiple ways to hear the topic described in different contexts (YouTube videos, ask professors for alternative explanations, actually read your textbook or First Aid).

Hosting group study sessions on specific topics may also help you decipher, articulate, and understand the language on in-house, and more importantly, Step exams.

For example, knowing the difference between "neoplasm", "cancer", "lesion", and "tumor" will help you understand and decode pathological concepts.

Understanding the clinical context in which words are used and why they are used will also help you encode/learn information more effectively.

Obstacle #3 | Not knowing where to start when you're lost:

When you're stuck on a topic/concept, the first step to figuring out what clarifying questions to ask or resources to find is understanding what types of questions the information you're learning will help you answer. Here are a few examples of this:

> ### What you learn in med school should help you...
>
> - identify specific steps of a pathway or mechanism (e.g. cause, effects, and everythang in between)
>
> - apply the knowledge of steps in a pathway to clinical situations and pharmaceutical interventions
>
> - visually and descriptively identify anatomical and cellular structures
>
> - understand how lab values and represent functions of the body
>
> - identify and explain exceptions to a rule or theory
>
> - identify a rare detail of a common disease (and vice versa)
>
> - know the most likely or least likely outcome of a clinical situation
>
> - make connections between other pathways and body systems

This list was derived from Bloom's Taxonomy of Learning (meaning this is what your professors use to generate learning objectives and questions. You're welcome.)

If you know which of these areas you are struggling with when learning a concept, it'll be easier to see where your mental gaps are and how you might fill them in.

Obstacle #4 | Not knowing how to apply the information you learn:
PRACTICE QUESTIONS! These can iron out all the kinks in your problem-solving process. This is equivalent to a *hard mark* in the dance world—when you practice as if it's showtime. You'll surprise yourself each time you think you got a question right, when you find out that you were looking at the question incorrectly.

Let practice questions humble you like this as much as possible BEFORE the test, while you can still learn from your mistakes.

After completing a set of practice questions, do a thorough review of the questions you got right AND wrong, while you have your lecture notes or materials open.

Also, updating your notes accordingly to track the completeness of your understanding will increase the benefits of doing and learning from practice questions.

Obstacle #5 | Trouble sifting through dense material and or identifying "high-yield" points:
Almost every lecture should come with a list of learning objectives (LOs) at the beginning (yes, the ones you usually skip). You should try to prioritize these items when studying.

Test questions are often generated from learning objectives, so if you don't pay attention to anything else, make sure you're able to answer and understand these. LOs can also be used to guide your note-taking or review sessions.

Also, comprehensive board preparation materials (e.g. Pathoma or First Aid, which I'll get to later on *pg. 40*) can help you figure out what you should prioritize when you study.

Obstacle #6 | Forgetting details:
Choose a method whether it's online flashcards, physical flashcards, spaced repetition (discussed right after this), or any other system that improves active recall to memorize the little details. Anki is a crowd-fav for this method.

Anki
I had no idea what this was going into medical school so I'll just assume that

you don't know about it either.

Anki (some people say 'ahn-kee' and others say 'ayng-kee', doesn't matter) is a form of spaced repetition. It's an app that will show you flashcards in an order and frequency that increases your long-term memory of the facts on each flashcard.

Disclaimer: This is in no way, an official Anki summary because I'm not an "ankier". In fact, I still have a love-hate relationship with Anki, because I find it helpful for some subjects and not as helpful for others. Reach out to the upperclassmen at your school or watch tutorials on YouTube to get a better feel of how this app works before you rule it in/out.

If you decide to become a part of Ankiland, a good place to start is downloading pre-made card decks that have the information that will be on Step. You can also download a bunch of add-ons (like ones that postpone cards, which come in handy when you skip a few days).

You can also add extra cards to the pre-made decks (that don't quite cover everything you're taught). To get the most out of this method,

unlock new cards (represented by the blue number) and see reviewed cards (the orange number) every day you learn new material so you aren't overwhelmed by all of the details you're expected to know. You can even sync your cards on all your devices, which makes it convenient for studying while you walk or work out at the gym.

Obstacle #7 | Wearing out methods that work. One method may not fit all.
Anki may work well for micro, but not for anatomy. Learning hematology may require you to do more practice questions to understand it, while endocrinology may require you to think more conceptually.

Try creating a game plan for each type of class (anatomy, biochemistry, pathophysiology, etc.) and tweak each sub-method until you find both general and specific methods that work for learning anything that is thrown at you.

Overcoming these obstacles will build your arsenal of buckets (to keep the hydrant theme going) and mental tools to solve many different types of complex problems.

Designing the Buckets: The Evolution of Your Study Style

As I mentioned before, finding a study method that works will be frustrating at first, and you may feel like you are putting in hours and hours of effort without getting results on practice questions, quizzes, or your first few tests. It's okay; it's part of the process. If you stick with what works and quickly get rid of what does not, it will all come together if you don't give up. Keeping an open mind to *how* you learn is the key to developing an effective study method that best fits you.

To give you an idea of what I mean, here's a peek into how my notes evolved into my own unique learning tool throughout first year:

The Evolution of My Study Style: A Visual Guide

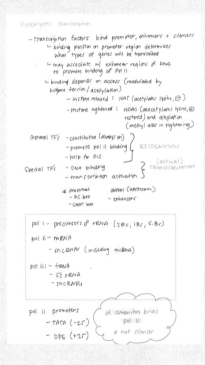

I was a big note-taker in college and for the MCAT, so I began med school taking notes *ad nauseam*—on the iPad, with actual paper, and even on my laptop. This wasn't effective AT ALL because each lecturer had their own set of notes which accomplished the same thing. My notes on ONE TOPIC would take up about THREE pages on average. It looked "nice" and organized, but it was not practical and I did not retain a thing.

< Here is a page of my Biochemistry Notes from Test Cycle (TC) 1

Then, I started to only prioritize taking notes on and or diagraming high-yield topics.

I slowly started to feel comfortable pulling info from multiple lectures together to create the big picture physically and mentally using "mind maps" and process diagrams.

Here is a page of my Biochemistry Notes from TC2 >

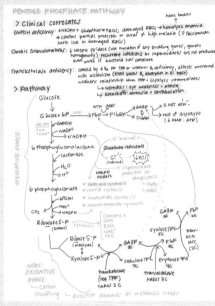

To take it to the next level, I completely left out unnecessary details in my notes. I knew that what I was excluding was "unnecessary" if it wasn't absolutely essential to understanding the bigger picture of the topic at hand. I left those unnecessary values, reference ranges, and straight facts for Anki, Quizlets, or other flashcards/ methods that solely strengthened rote memorization. The types of diagrams I ended up making took many forms including:

Tree diagrams
This one is from the Musculoskeletal block

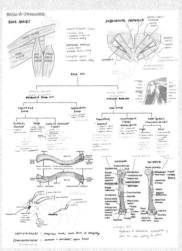

Algorithms

This one is from the Hematology/ Immunology block

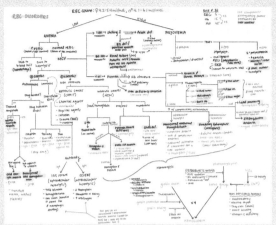

Mind Maps

This one is also from the Hematology and Immunology block.

(This includes all of the major physiology concepts covered for the whole block.)

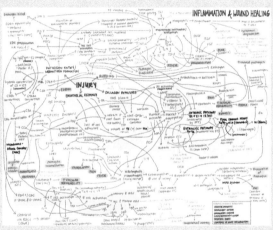

Pictograms

Anatomy, TC3

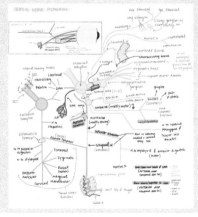

Hybrid diagrams

(with multiple diagramming styles depending on the body system)
Endocrinology Block

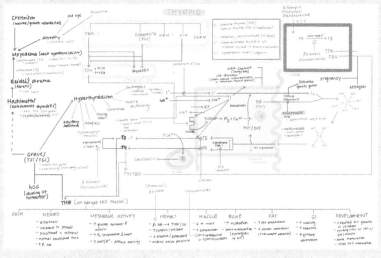

All made with GoodNotes for iPad

Before you panic, I did NOT make a diagram for every topic, or even for every high yield topic. Instead, I used diagramming as a learning tool for the topics most important to understanding each body system as a whole. I rarely used these diagrams to review, but as a reference to how I processed the information I learned.

In other words, the diagrams gave me a birds-eye view of what I grasped from lectures. This also helped me visualize gaps in my knowledge,

which then guided my review and application of the information.

Also, they were a guilt-free creative outlets that were just so pretty to look at when I was done! So I liked this method for that reason too.

Although this method was very pain-staking and took a lot of time, it worked for ME and made me a more effective learner. My expectation is NOT that this strategy will also work for you, but that you'll understand how limitless the possibilities are for how unique your learning method and styles can be. So, if the learning styles "myth" doesn't cut it for you, no worries.

TO THE DRAWING BOARD WE GO!

Customizing Your Study Style: The Blueprint

No matter how many unique methods there are, every sturdy study style boils down to these five elements:

You can use this outline to create or modify your style.

- **Time:** How much time do you have to study? To take breaks in between? Is this enough? If not, do you pre-read, watch lectures ahead of time, or front load your week? *(pg. 38)*

- **Focus:** How will you get in and stay in your study zone? *(pg. 38)*

- **Efficiency:** You don't have all day to study, so what encoding strategies and tricks will you use to make the most out of your study time? *(see obstacles starting on pg. 28 for more on this)*

- **Progress Tracking:** What is your signal that you've covered as much as you can? Is it the number of practice questions? Is it the number of lectures you can get done in a day?

- **Review:** *This is often overlooked but is just as important as the others, if not more.* How do you know that you can recall AND apply everything you learned? *(see below)*

Customizing Your Study Style: Flesh it out! *(all derived from source 1)*

Now that you have the barebones of how your style might look, here are some effective, evidence-based tools that can help it come to life:

Interleaving

Study biochem for an hour, then micro, then anatomy, then path, then circle back to biochem. This is more helpful than staring at 1000 anatomy slides straight.

You'd be surprised how many connections this method helps you make between different subjects. You can even do a set of practice questions that cover multiple subjects at once. *Interleaving keeps it spicy.*

Elaboration (sometimes referred to as *elaborative integration*) When learning a topic, don't just try to memorize the bare minimum.

Make all of the connections you can between the piece of information you want to learn and things you already know or are currently learning in other classes.

I promise that when you learn or review related information months later, it won't be as overwhelming. Plus, the connections you make now will be gold once you review (and relearn) this information for boards. Do the most upfront; you'll be glad you did in the long run.

Self-explanation

This is my favorite. If you can't teach it or explain it, you don't know it. Don't just recite a fact that you know, but push yourself to mentally recall everything you know about a concept and explain why it makes sense. This is your chance to channel your inner five-year-old: keep asking "why" until you get answers.

If you don't know where to start when answering these mental prompts, especially for the concepts that are heavy-hitters for boards, that's a red flag. But if you practice this and master it, you'll rely less on straight, rote memorization to learn—which is ideal for board prep.

Active recall

This may be the most uncomfortable thing to do, but it works. Actively test yourself on each topic as much as you possibly can, even the ones that you remember or understand the least.

Grab a study partner and have them quiz you. Dust off your practice question book and do some random questions on the information you've covered to test how well you can retrieve the info.

Dual encoding

Maximize the number of ways the information is stored in your mind. After days of learning from a textbook, switch it up by watching a lecture or an animated 3-D model of the concepts you're learning. (When using this strategy, make sure you don't become resource overloaded).

If I'm keepin' it a buck with ya, how you study early on in the game matters. This is because you WILL see all of this stuff in a year or so on boards. So as you start thinking about how you'll tackle and soak up information, adopt methods that will help you learn for the long term.

Your Study Schedule

After choosing a unique study style, the time you will need to put this plan in motion should become more clear. Sometimes it doesn't, and that's okay too. When you figure out how much time you need, stick to that number.

"Okay, but Ja'Neil seriously, how much time should I spend studying?"

Instead of a number, I'll give you a word that I will keep repeating until you get it. The word is EFFICIENCY. Some people study all day, but if you don't need to, DON'T DO IT.

However, to find a happy medium, you may need to try studying material until you're exhausted, and or try doing the bare minimum to see how your performance changes. It's also helpful to know your

curriculum (pass/fail vs graded, and the minimum passing score for tests and classes) so you can determine how much effort/support/rest you'll need to get a score you're satisfied with.

Unfortunately, there is no hack for this but, you have the entire year to troubleshoot this process. Trust me, all of this planning will pay off when you need it the most. You got this!

Finding & Staying in Your Study Groove

After you overcome the obstacles of learning lecture material and coming up with a study schedule, you may find it hard to have a productive hour or two studying the info. It happens to the best of us.

However, if you want to stay in your study groove for a few hours, there are many ways to get into the zone:

The Prodromo Method
This is a popular way to maximize break time and productivity time. This study method consists of alternating timed study bursts and study breaks.

It works by breaking up your study time into twenty-five-minute uninterrupted work chunks and five-minute breaks.

Each interval is called a prodromo. One prodromo consists of one work chunk and one break chunk. After four or five of these, you should increase your break chunks until they equal your work chunks.

My Modified Prodomo Method

I personally do not benefit from twenty-five-minute study intervals and can spend at least twenty-five minutes just to get into the full swing of my study sessions. For me, a three-hour session of uninterrupted work is my sweet spot for effective studying.

So, I take proportional breaks in between each work chunk: for each hour, I take ten minutes to break. So for example, after studying for three hours straight, I take a thirty-minute break.

You can alter or modify either method as you see fit, but brain breaks are a must.

Drowning Out the World: Curating a Productivity Playlist

Before med school, I heard about surgeons who played classical music in the operating room to concentrate. It's called the *Mozart Effect*. And for a long time, I didn't believe the hype. Also, I— having a background in music theory and vocal performance—thought it was impossible to listen to a song without not paying attention to or appreciating all of its elements (the baseline, the chords, the motifs, etc.). *How could art be background noise?*

However, once I tried listening to some jazz classics during my study time, I was amazed at how focused I was. It worked like magic. In addition to jazz, there are a bunch of genres that can get you into grind mode:

- Classical orchestral music
- Baroque classical music
- Classical piano solos
- Big band jazz
- Cool jazz
- Classic funk
- Cinematic music
- Electronic
- Instrumental alternative R&B

If none of these genres float your boat, try finding music that meets these criteria:

How to Pick the Right Study Bops

- rhythmic instrumental music or music with minimal lyrics (ideally lyrics or song titles with an uplifting message)

- songs without a loud top layer (e.g. music without a noticeable high-hat or snare drum beat) or songs with a prominent baseline

- songs with repetitive verses, choruses, or vamps

- music between 70-90 beats per minute (bpm)

- compositions with different textural layers (e.g. clickers or a deep bongo drum)

Drowning Out the World: "Creating" Silence

Remember those noise-canceling earphones I suggested earlier? These can help you get into your grind mode wherever you are.

Those distractions gotta go!

If you know that your phone is enemy #1 for your study time, TURN IT OFF. Or put it on DND. Putting a time limit on social media apps works too.

If your friends are enemies #2-4, but give you comfort and support during studying, alternate between group and solo study days. At the end of the day, you will be taking your exams by yourself, so make sure group study helps more than it hurts.

Comfort is not always key

Studying in your bed is a trap. If that is your only choice, "de-comfortize" (you heard it here first) your bed and get a lap desk. You can't afford to subconsciously associate sleep with studying. Remember, there's so much info to cover in such little time.

Must-Have Med School Resources

There is a wealth of resources out there (some of which are FREE), so don't feel pressured to purchase all of your required texts unless it is necessary.

When sampling resources:
- Check with upperclassmen to see what worked for them, why, and how they used them.
- Try a variety of flashcards, videos, podcasts, hard copies, & eBooks.
- Avoid becoming volume overloaded. Settle on a solid three or four resources that you work for you.

Here are some of the OG resources that were helpful for me during my first year:

- **First Aid:** This tells you EVERYTHING you need to know (you'll frequently hear the phrase "high yield" to describe this important info) about what will be tested on your Step 1 exam that will take place in your second year.

  If you annotate this resource throughout your first two years, you'll be ahead by the time it's time to study boards.

  It also has an appendix with a chart that ranks and grades other helpful study resources.

- **Costanzo Physiology:** This book has in-depth descriptions of high-yield physio topics for every body system.

- **Fundamentals of Pathology:** The pathology bible. Written by Hussain A. Sattar.

- **A Solid Question Bank:** *Board Review Series*, BRS Physiology (also written by Costanzo), and *Gray's Anatomy Review* are my favorite resources for practice questions. They both offer bite-sized reviews of high-yield information and have a bunch of board-style questions with explanations.

- **A Solid Anatomy Atlas:** *Netter's Complete Anatomy Atlas* is my fav and helped me understand the context of the structures I was learning about in lecture and seeing in the lab.

- **Additional Study Aid Subscriptions** (when your lectures fail you, these won't):
  - SketchyMedical- Videos that give you fun stories (like the ones I mentioned in the learning curve section) to remember pathophys concepts. It's also good for learning

drugs and microbiology (which is what I used it for).

- **Picmonic-** An additional visual learning aid for drugs and micro. Has more content than Sketchy.
- **Pixorize-** Alternative for above source. Their video quality is top tier.
- **Amboss-** Includes up-to-date expert content reviews and practice questions
- **U World-Rx -** A question bank with great boards-style questions and explanations
- **Boards and Beyond-** Great videos for basic physiology; the condensed version of the high-yield info you need to know for boards

- **YouTube (FREEEE):** I plan on dedicating my medical degree to:
  - Ninja Nerd- For all of your physiology needs. He breaks difficult topics down into their bits and pieces and explains them all clearly. His videos are worth watching all the way through

because he dumbs everything down so you can understand the concepts backward and forward. *If I could marry him, I would.*

- Medicosis Perfectionalis- This guy is hilarious and has great visuals to help memorize concepts. He is also good at comparing similar topics (e.g. Lymphoma vs Leukemia)
- Arnando Hasudungan- His drawings are awesome. He doesn't go in-depth into minor physio details but explains major concepts in a way that sticks.
- MedCram- This source came onto the scene later on in my first year, but I wish I had known about it sooner. They do an amazing job at breaking large clinical applications down into understandable chunks.

- **Databases:** *Up-to-Date*, is a medical website that includes the most updated protocols and standards for patient care— physical exam maneuvers, standard values and limits, best practices, etc. Another great peer-reviewed resource is *PubMed*, which Google will start to suggest when it finds out you're in medical school. These databases may be more relevant in M3, but it's still good to know they exist.

Emptying the Buckets: Test-Taking Strategies

If you've made it this far to med school, you have taken what may have felt like the hardest test of your life, the MCAT. If I'm being honest here, that may be one of the easiest tests you ever will from this point forward.

You remember those tertiary questions right? The ones where they didn't flat out ask you to identify a structure, but asked you to figure out what the patient in the question had, understand how to identify the relevant values, plug them into an equation, and then use the answer you got to finally match it to the right answer choice? Yea, those really hard

questions within the question. It's inception for med students. Getting super comfortable with solving problems to this degree is the key to acing your in-house and board-style test questions.

Yea, I know this may seem like a huge mountain to climb, but believing that you can do this, despite the minor setbacks, will get you further than pulling a bunch of all-nighters during test week.

Grounding techniques, mantras, and test-taking strategies matter and can make the difference when you're on the verge of having a panic attack while sitting in front of the exam paper (or screen). I'll mention a few of mine in just a few, but if all else fails:

NEVER start a test with doubts that you won't ace it. That is half the battle.

Decode & translate to divide & conquer

Correctly answering a question begins with decoding, defining, and identifying all of the keywords in the question stem and the answer choices. This is another reason why it's helpful to know as much medical jargon as possible.

Own the first minute

During tests, I tend to easily remember most of the overarching concepts. However, with only a few minutes left on the exam, I may forget the specific variables in Fick's equation or forget the numerical blood pressure range for primary vs secondary hypertension, etc.

Exam test fatigue may also prevent you from recalling key details when your brain starts to get tired. If this is your struggle, dedicate the first minute of the test to taking a deep breath and pouring all of the relevant equations and concept models you remember onto your scrap paper—even before looking at the first question. Writing details out first may be worth trying if this is a weak point in your test-taking strategy.

Boost your confidence & save time

Another problem you may have is running out of time to answer every question. For the exams that don't allow you to go back and review questions (Anatomy practicals for example), you will just have to think fast or practice differently by maximizing active recall methods (flashcards/visual aids).

More commonly, on the exams that allow you to navigate back and forth between questions, give all of the questions a first pass, answer the ones you know off the top of your head, and skip/ flag the ones that are a bit tougher.

This method does two things: It boosts your confidence about the amount of information you know while also suppressing the fear of not knowing enough to pass the exam. Both may help you ride out the initial nervousness associated with starting the exam and give you extra time to focus on tougher questions.

Follow your gut

There will always be two answers that seem right, and you will always be stuck between two. Step questions are also like this. Go with your gut (based on what you studied *for real*). Reason out why one is wrong. Never guess. *And again, remember to breathe.*

Once you've convinced yourself that an answer choice is correct, DO NOT change it. I can't tell you how many times I got a question wrong because I changed it at the last second to the incorrect option.

Track your flags

Being present during exams is my secret sauce. Remembering the feelings of being unsure vs. confidently knowing answers (from my practice question sessions) allows me to pretty accurately predict how many questions I get right/wrong on an exam. Some say it's a gift. I call it a little strategy and mindfulness.

Using the flagging tool on tests helps me take advantage of this "gift".

For you, it may help you create mental notes about the type or number of questions you're unsure about. Either way, mastering this skill is key. Not just to help you estimate what score you will get, but so you know how much command you have (or do not have) over the test material.

Learning how to gauge your mistakes will help you become a better test taker. It will also help you see patterns in your thought process during exams to guide the pace of your study routine.

Physical Diagnosis & OSCEs

Objective Structured Clinical Examination, or OSCEs for short, are timed exams that assess your clinical skills—taking blood pressure, completing a thorough patient interview, using ultrasound equipment, palpating, percussing (tapping), and auscultating (listening to) deeper structures in the body not visible from the outside. You'll take a series of OSCEs at the end of each year.

In preparation for these, you'll likely take a class called PDx (which is short for physical diagnosis). This is the traditional way to develop your "doctoring" skills and to finally apply all of the facts and information you learn in lecture to live patients.

Watch and learn

First, check to see what your school's passing standard is for each OSCE (down to the tee). *Bates Visual Examination Guide* was recommended by my school as a visual aid to help me learn how to perform the different exams. They also have a book with the directions in plain text. Check with your school to see if there is a specific guide that you should reference.

YouTube, once again, is gold. *Drs Manual* is a free channel that demonstrates physical exam maneuvers.

OLD CAARTS at ROSs need SOAP

The best ways to get a hang of these skills are to stick to a systematic approach and get into a routine.

Staged/real patients won't tell you the key, "buzzword" signs and symptoms you usually see in question stems. It's up to you to determine what details of the interview/physical exam helps to paint a full clinical picture. *(if you were ever wondering what really separates physicians from other doctors, this is it, my friend)*

"OLD CAARTS at ROSs need SOAP" is one way to remember all of the important parts of the history & physical exam (H&P). It also outlines how most physicians structure most patient interviews.

SOAP-Subjective, Objective, Assessment, Plan:

Subjective-The **story** the patient will give you about their condition and their current/past medical history. The subjective story includes

"**OLD CAARTS**" (onset, location on the body, duration, character/ type of pain, associated symptoms, alleviating/ aggravating factors, radiation, time course, pain severity). The subjective also includes **"ROSs"**: the review of systems. It's a detailed inventory of each possible symptom related to each body system and is obtained via a series of questions and yes/no answers. In other words, it's a patient's head-to-toe self-report of their body systems. *The ROS catches any other symptoms not discussed in the OLD CAARTS that are equally important to reaching an accurate diagnosis.*

For example, in a cardiovascular (CV) ROS, you might ask the patient if they're experiencing heartburn, chest pain, palpitations (feeling like their heart is beating fast), shortness of breath, leg swelling, blood clots, enlarged veins, or leg cramping. All of these are indicators of CV function.

Other parts of the subjective include medications, allergies, travel history, medical/surgical history, family medical history, social history, sexual history, and spiritual history— all of which have their own structure/sections.

Another skill you'll develop is knowing which questions to ask (or not ask) to efficiently gather the information you need while you also engage with the patient.

Objective- The **optics** of the patient; physical exam (lung/ heart sounds, reflexes, etc.) findings only. This is where your clinical skills practice time comes into play.

Assessment- How will you tie **ALL** of the information from the encounter together? What does all the information you gathered mean? What might the patient have? How will you communicate this to the patient?

Plan- What are the next steps? Meds? Procedures? Follow-up?

There's a ton of mnemonics you can use to help you navigate an H&P. Try a few different ones or even make your own!

Practice is key
No matter how these skills are taught during required PDx classes, you will have to put in extra time to master them. With learning these skills— and everything else in first year for that matter—it may seem like you do not know what you are doing half of the time, and you might feel like you are just aimlessly going through the motions. But this is literally what medical school is for. If there is ever a time to mess up and confess that you don't know what you're doing and why, this is the time. No one is a natural at this stuff. And if it seems like a lot of people are, they're most likely faking it, or have put in extra time to get it right. Hey, I failed my first OSCE, and I live to tell the story. So, handle your business and ace those OSCEs. You got this.

Getting Help to Carry the Buckets: Academic Support

A Word on Tutors
Before the word, "tutor" sends you onto a mental tangent about all the reasons why you don't need one, hear me out. Prior to med school, I had been literally at the top of my class since fifth grade. I had always adjusted to the academic bar when it was raised and was fine. I was your typical straight-A student. I had a tutor one time in fifth grade and it was pointless.

However, the endocrinology block in February of first year sent me into panic mode when I realized that rote memorization wouldn't work for this body system (or for the long-term memorization of anything I learned so far). So after being completely lost the first week of that block, I decided to apply for a student tutor through my school.

Was the tutor teaching me the information? No. My tutor taught me how to conceptualize information instead of just memorizing it. So although this notion of getting a tutor might seem aimless, it wouldn't hurt to get a tutor during your first year while you're still trying to get your bearings on a study method that works for you. *You don't get extra credit for figuring it out all on your own.*

Educational Consultants

They are specialists who are trained to help you try strategies (diagramming, mind mapping, methods of spaced repetition) to enhance your learning. Ask if your school if you have access to one. You'd be surprised how much may be available to you through the dean's office. Whatever you decide, DO NOT suffer in silence. It is possible to do well no matter the means to get there.

THE BOTTOM LINE(S)

No matter how you look at it, you have to know everything you're taught in your first and second year.

Some days, you'll feel the brunt of the hydrant effect. But no need to fear. It's not really about what you learn, but *how* you learn that will make or break your learning experience. **Hack your brain.**

When trying to adjust your study styles and test-taking strategies, make sure that you are always able to **visualize the big picture** of the topic at hand. You will easily get burnt out if all you do is memorize details.

Adopting strategies that will help you **balance conceptualization and active recall** methods will maximize your capacity to memorize, retain, and apply information, and will give you the confidence to ace your in-house and standardized tests.

Most importantly, if you're struggling to find strategies that work, **reach out for help** before it's too late!

Additional Resources

1. "What Works, What Doesn't", J. Dunlonsky, K. Rawson, E.J. Marsh, M. J. Nathan, and D. Willingham; published in the *Scientific American Mind*, 2013 issue.

How to Study in Medical School, 2nd Edition—Armin Kamyab

section 3
The Art of Doctah-ing it Up:
Growing Into the Role of "Doctor"

You may have been wondering how I chose the title of this book. Just imagine for a second, my mom saying the phrase in the thickest patwah-tinged New York accent you can imagine. She said it to describe how she adds her special spices and secret ingredients— you know, the ones that are never measured— to recipes to make them tasty.

In my first year, she used the phrase to describe how I'm adding my own dash of personality to this journey to become the best doctah I can be.

Thanks, mom.

"Standards" of Professionalism

Contrary to popular belief, there is no universal standard for medical professionalism. Yes, be polite, considerate, and on time. Yes, respect your superiors. Yes, be aware of your influence and who you represent. Yes, dress according to the contracts you signed. But outside of that, professionalism is subjective, which leaves a lot of room for your unique personality and experiences to frame your development into a physician.

On my first day of class, I felt like everything different about me was magnified by 100%, and it was clear that I was not in Jersey anymore. It was August 2020, I could count the number of black girls on my hand, and I looked around the lecture hall and wondered if my clothes were too "loud". I even felt the vibes change when I introduced myself to my new classmates as an HBCU alum.

Although being the racial minority was an obvious difference, it was my entire persona that didn't seem to fit the nerdy, privileged, cis-gender, older-white male image of "doctor" I was fed my whole life (and filled the seats of the lecture hall around me).

Don't get me wrong, I did not think about this all of the time but stepping into the world of medical academia often emphasized the contrast between it and *my* "world". It also made me realize how I was currently changing the face of physicianship just by being me; and that I couldn't continue to do so if all I did was trade in who I was in for a white coat. So, you may be thinking, *"What does this all have to do with professionalism?"* Well, everything.

My experience was an example of the internal battle that happens during the passage into physicianhood. Undergrad may not have exposed your lack of empathy, required you to wear a pressed shirt, or forced you to see the consequences of your learning efforts be so closely linked to another person's (a patient's) life and well-being.

This stage is a tricky one because medicine is not just a field, it is a culture. As a result, adopting doctor-like characteristics can be a life-changing experience—especially when the standard set before you looks completely different from what/who you are. Plus, when grades and evaluations that are the currency of approval are attached to this identity, it's sometimes easier to choose this new standard of acting and thinking over your past self—which *is* the point of higher education. But at what cost?

So, I started medical school, raw and fresh-faced. Soon after, I noticed that my jokes didn't hit the same, my tolerance for over-explaining cultural references vanished, and I started saying things I'd never heard before like "tattered", "concomitant", and, my fav, "in a pickle". And more than just changing for maturity's or education's sake, pieces of my identity and culture started to seem more palatable if watered down. And then there was this back and forth, between the monotonous, concrete person I was at school and the artsy, free person I was at home. Then, I started to spend more time at school, and then who I really was got less airtime. The identity of the student I was expected to be and the person I was raised to be were at odds. It is this constant opposition that—aside from being the recipe for textbook code-switching—fueled my obsession with finding a way to be 100% me and 100% doctor. (Pardon my math.)

This struggle may not be present or extreme for everyone (or you). One camp could care less about keeping their personal and professional selves separate. Others seem to be stubbornly determined to blend both identities into one. Just in case it's not already obvious, I share the latter sentiment and believe that the world of medicine needs you to be your authentic self and a doctor at the same time. I'm convinced that it's necessary and possible. *Medical school is a time to be molded, not carved down to someone you're not.*

In other words, **your standard of professionalism should be a mix of the best of who you are and what is required for you to advance in this field.**

So, when determining what kind of student or physician you want to be, ask yourself, "how important is it for who I am to shine?"

When to Speak Up: Navigating Sensitive Conversations

Now, of course, the standard you choose does not change where you are on the medical food chain (*see the hierarchy on pg. 110*). Even though the culture of medicine has evolved, you gotta remember that there is still a lot of work to be done so that the spectrum of standards I speak of is universally accepted.

So, if you, a first-year, a minority of any kind maybe, hear a seasoned attending, —especially one who is "ol' school"—make an ignorant comment, think about how responding to the comment (if you choose to) would represent or misrepresent your standard.

Fighting words vs. Feedback
Another thing to consider is if the comment was fighting words or feedback.

This journey, like any other professional track, will increase your threshold for things that may normally rub you the wrong way. Knowing this limit will save you a lot of heartache from reacting to or tolerating every negative encounter of your med school experience. Sometimes business *is* business and criticism is not always personal.

Feedback is constructive, supportive, enhances your learning process, encourages growth, and is necessary.

Feedback can also take the form of environmental cues that you can use to determine how much you will tolerate as a student physician.

Maybe all of the staff on that floor play strictly by the book, or maybe unpacking the doctor's comment with only one day left isn't worth it this time.

Fighting words, however, are targeted, rooted in prejudice, are based on assumptions, perpetuate close-mindedness, and are unnecessary.

Maybe this is the third time Dr. F commented on your hijab, and the third time it has disrupted your focus and learning experience.

Either of these may be uncomfortable to receive, but can both be opportunities for you to grow as a professional and a communicator. If you find yourself in a difficult conversation with a superior, whatever you do, don't pop off, and make sure you take a moment to process the situation (whether you respond in real-time, at a later date, or vent to a friend or trusted colleague). Never hold it in.

When responding to offensive comments, phrases that start with "At this moment I felt..." and "I noticed that..." usually do the trick.

Wait, how is this different from code-switching? What happened to authenticity? Glad you asked.

Clear communication is universal. This tool is the best way you can advocate for yourself and is the only way that the professional culture of medicine can improve.

I realize that this may be a big ask because having these hard conversations on the reg is emotionally draining—especially when comments are targeted at a group or belief with which you identify.

But hear me out, every time you correct microaggressions and comments that don't "sit right" on the receiving end, you are not just speaking for yourself.

You are sometimes correcting traditions of flawed thinking that impact the learning and healing environments of future students, clinicians, and patients.

To be completely honest, I dropped the ball where this is concerned in my first year. There were times when I was too passive because I lacked "the perfect words" to say what I felt, or was triggered to the point where I couldn't even get words out. But it's okay, because speaking up takes practice.

It is an art.

So as I am requiring this of myself, I'm also advising you to give yourself grace as you find out what your standard is, and how to mean what you say and say what you mean.

Also, don't just act like the nurse if they mistakenly call you one. And lastly, PLEASE correct those who mispronounce your name.

A few words for allies (of any kind):

- It is easier than you think to operate under the influence of your biases
- It only takes a spark to gaslight
- Martyrizing allyship defeats its purpose
- The bliss of ignorance is the ugly cousin to the discomfort of change
- It should never be the sole responsibility of the oppressed to stop their oppression
- Be aware of your privilege so you can use it for good.
  Please and thanks.

You are a professional in training with a whole white coat. You'll soon be one of the most respected professionals in the world, so know that your name and your words have weight (whether you like it or not).

What you say and do from here on out has power, and can influence the culture of medicine for the better. But of course, no pressure.

The Questions You Aren't Obligated to Answer

Unfortunately, the majority of uncomfortable conversations you'll have during first year will occur amongst your classmates. The ugly truth is that medical school is competitive, even in pass/fail programs. People, as innocent as they may seem, *will* find new ways to get you to talk about your grades or petty drama (yes, even at this level).

You'll even have some gunners (*see glossary*) mention their grades or ranking to breed competition. Don't fall into the trap. Competition is not a good look and is the opposite of the spirit of professionalism.

The following questions, although frequently asked, have NOTHING to do with how good of a med student you are or how good of a doctor you will become. You shouldn't feel pressured to answer any of these (yes, even when asked by attendings) if you don't want to, no matter how "friendly" the conversation may seem:

"What was your MCAT score?"

It was good enough for you to get into med school, even if it was by the skin of your teeth. No matter what kind of student you were in the past, what your score was, or what your GPA was, it is just as possible for you to kill the game in first year as it is for the person who got a 520. It is also very possible that the "520-ers" in your class struggle just as much — if not more — as you might be. So don't sweat it.

Past scores and grades aside, you can still be very successful in medical school. Listen here, since you hit the accept button, the playing field of opportunity has been leveled.

"What was your major?"

Again, there is often a little shade thrown to those who didn't major in biology during undergrad. And I still don't understand why.

If you are among those who had a non-traditional major before starting med school, you should be proud of that, and nothing less. Cookie-cutter credentials are boring and don't count for much once you make it to med school. If anything, depending on what your major was, you'll be able to relate to your patients in more unique ways than most of your classmates.

So no, you may have not taken anatomy or histo, but you are just as capable of learning the material well. In the wise words of every Jamaican aunt who has come before me, *don't let nobody tek yuh fi eddiat.*

"What specialty are you interested in?"

If you know, great! But if you don't, it's totally fine. You don't even know what parts of medicine you like or don't like because you haven't seen jack yet (ask any third-year on rotations). Figuring this out is what medical school is for. You're likely to change what you want to specialize in five or so times anyway. You should simply know your interests but keep an open mind and stay curious.

"Are you here on a scholarship?"

I gotta be honest, it is very likely that I received a full-ride to medical school because of affirmative action. The ad com at my school would not have selected me if I wasn't a strong applicant. However, I know that my race was heavily weighed to reflect my school's intentional push for diversity, equity, and inclusion. Which is great! But to many, this is seen as a handout. It took everything within me to not let that overshadow the fact that, besides me being black, I am also smart, driven, and talented.

So, if you don't want to tell people about your scholarship, don't. Let your authentic self prove why you deserve to be in medical school.

And if you got a full scholarship, love that for you. Just remember that it's a privilege to be in your shoes, not a reason to think you are better than the person in the next pair.

"Do you have any publications?"

Trust me, half of my classmates got into med school without any publications (like me), research experience, or shadowing. Don't feel bad if you haven't authored a publication yet. You have access to so many professors and PIs who'd love to have med students like you work in their labs and get published.

"What did you get on that test?"

I strongly suggest that you avoid answering this question like the Bubonic plague. Your grades are like your Amazon password and your debit-card pin—you can't trust everyone with them. Only share your scores with those who have your best interest in mind (true friends, mentors, tutors, etc.)

If you're itching to know how well you're doing compared to your classmates, or if you're on the right track to match into the specialty you are considering, talk to your academic advisor or dean.

Assuming Leadership Roles

For some reason, finding clubs and initiatives to be a part of is rarely a problem for us med students. The hardest part might be saying "no" so you don't stretch yourself too thin.

Hate to break it to you (once again), but I have attended quite a few match panels during match season—where fourth years talk about the match process. Many residency directors who attended revealed while your roles as class president or class advisors for clubs are important, they can mean very little to residency programs if they are just resume boosters.

So if you want to be involved in a position or office during your first year (amongst all of the things you will have on your plate) make sure that it is not just there to make you look good on paper. Be involved in things that will make your med school experience unique and one-of-a-kind.

Choose roles that highlight your leadership skills (even if you're growing into them) and positions that highlight the most amazing parts of who you are.

For example, I was super passionate about mentorship before starting med school (as you can probably tell by now). So, both of my current positions allow me to be a mentor and resource for pre-meds in ways that use creative combinations of mixed media content.

Med School Clubs & Honor Societies You'll Want to Be a Part of
Here are some nationally recognized organizations that you can be a part of in your first year and beyond:

- American Medical Association- Medical Student Section (AMA-MSS)
- American Medical Student Association (AMSA)
- American Medical Women's Association- Student Division (AMWA)
- Latino Medical Student Association (LMSA)
- Student National Medical Association (SNMA)

Alpha Omega Alpha (AOA) is a national honor society for medical school students. Depending on your chapter requirements, eligibility may be determined based on GPA, rank, average test grade, amount of high honors, or recommendations you may receive from your school's chapter committee members and board. Students are selected to apply by their school's committee in their third or fourth year.

Gold Humanism Honor Society (GHHS) is another honor society. Membership can be achieved by peer nomination in your third year. The top 15% of nominees are distinguished as role models within their school's community based on compassion, professionalism, and service.

The Value of Research Projects

Although you may have faked that you liked research to apply for medical school, that is no longer the case. It is very important that this time around, you only do research if you want to; and if you do, choose labs/ subjects you're passionate about (and yes, it can be a topic/ thesis unrelated to basic science!).

Lemme say it this way: you don't have time to waste pipetting and logging in values if that's not your thing (this is your moment to take a sigh of relief). Nevertheless, if you

decide to work on a project, a coveted accomplishment will be to publish your research in a well-known research journal. Equally important is presenting your research at a major medical conference, research symposium, or poster competition. It's a way to show that even before you get your MD, you are doing what needs to be done to develop into a leader and trailblazer in the worlds of medicine and science.

Unlike summer research projects in undergrad, these projects don't have a definite start and end date. Also, keep in mind that clinical research is easier to publish than basic science research—which can take years of analyzing data. Please, I beg you, be strategic about which projects you start.

Your goals should be to contribute to/ learn from the research process and to produce publications, or "pubs" (abstracts, manuscripts, or poster presentations) so you can refer to them years down the line in interviews for residency. Research and any other contributions to medicine you make as a medical student are especially important if you are attending a school with a pass/fail curriculum. In addition to your grades and board scores, pubs will set you apart from other applicants. In addition to it being a great look on your CV, research projects are a great way to network with sub-specialists, create relationships with faculty, and make a bit of extra cash on the side. These things will come in handy later on when it's time to apply for residency, but will hurt you early on if you're only trying to pad your CV.

Research can be done at any time during your first year (*if* you have the time, which is rare), the summer after your first year (like I did), or any time before residency applications.

Once you express interest in a lab and get hired, check with your PI to see what publication type is appropriate for you to write.

Here are five examples of publication types you can author:

- **Original Research Article:** The classic type of article published in peer-reviewed journals (one that has been reviewed and approved by experts in a certain field).

This type of entry hypothesizes a new medical or science phenomenon and is supported by an **experiment** or analyzed data sets.

- **Case Report:** A write-up of a **unique clinical presentation** that can serve as a teaching point for medical diagnosis. A case series is a similar option that includes three or more unique cases.

- **Abstract:** A **qualitative** grouping of related published articles that support new or unique conclusions. Basically, a write-up that makes connections between existing journal articles.

- **Meta-Analysis:** It's the same thing as an abstract but instead of compiling the conclusions of articles, the author compiles and cross-references **quantitative (numerical)** data sets.

- **Op-Ed:** Short for "opposite the editorial page"; an essay that offers an **alternate opinion** to the author's intended argument in a journal article.

For a full list of publications types and characteristics, visit the NIH website.

A Word on Authorship

The PI (principal investigator; the person in charge of the lab, the boss) has the right to not list you as the first author of your work—even if you wrote and edited the abstract all by yourself— because it is their lab.

It is simply a part of medical and traditional research culture. So please don't get all in ya feelings if you see your name after theirs or after the name of the head research assistant.

If you are unsure of the authoring traditions in your lab, just ask. PIs understand that you are trying to be a competitive student and want to boost your CV. Talk to them about your concerns so you know where to expect to see your name on the authorship list.

Also, talk to people (Ph.D. or MD/Ph.D. students) who are familiar with that lab's culture to determine if that PI is right for you before committing.

After all, research is NOT a requirement

If you decide to not be a part of a research project during first year, or med school period IT IS OKAY.

Read that one more time. And again for good measure. Many people match into top programs without research/pubs. So, you don't have to engage in research, but it will only help you if you do.

Staying Connected to Your "Why"

You may not have time during first year for research projects, but there are many other ways to remain connected to the reasons why you started med school in the first place.

Shadowing Opportunities & Preceptorships

Around November of first year, I wasn't really feelin' med school and was of touch with my "why".

At my medical school, every student is assigned to a faculty mentor. So after telling my mentor about my dilemma, she told me that I could get up and walk right into the hospital at any time to shadow any willing physician I could find for inspiration.

The very next week, I did just that and shadowed her colleague in the pediatric (or peds for short) emergency department (ED) for a few hours. It was so cool to me that I could just randomly ask any type of doctor to follow them around, and that I had full ID access at the hospital. Now that I was a med student, the hospital was my "playground". Shadowing was a great way to take a break from looking at a screen all day to interact with patients, which is the end goal of this journey, anyways.

Signing up for a preceptorship is a more formal way of getting shadowing hours. This is a more structured experience with a physician-mentor who will give you personal advice, training, and guidance within their field.

Interest Groups

In addition to shadowing, school-associated interest groups are a great way to get exposure to certain specialties and sub-specialties. They are the best-kept secret when it comes to carving out your specific path to residency and beyond. Attending interest groups can provide you with research opportunities, internships, preceptorships, and more.

Grand Rounds

Hospital grand rounds are seminars that present medical cases and advances in in-patient care to an interdisciplinary audience including physicians, pharmacists, residents, and medical students.

This is a great way to stay connected to all of the new policies and discoveries in the world of medicine. I attended many of these in undergrad and it helped color my reality of what medicine might look like by the time I can practice it. Check with your dean's office or associated hospital admin to know when the next grand round will happen.

Journal Clubs

If you're into research, this may serve a similar purpose of staying up-to-date with all things medicine. Journal clubs are meetings where docs and student-docs meet to critically review published articles. They are usually specific to certain specialties, so if you are interested in a particular subset of medicine journal clubs might help you explore those interests.

Committees

Being an active member on a school board or committee is a great way to shape various aspects of the learning environment around you (professionalism, social events, curricula, resilience, wellness, etc.).

This is also a great opportunity to develop as a leader and a student advocate.

Community Involvement
Will you have time to be a volunteer in med school? Do community projects help you become a competent physician? Are residency programs actually interested to know that you enjoy giving back to your community? Yes, yes, and YES!

Being a community leader in nearby clinics, schools, and outreach programs is the most fulfilling way to develop humanity and compassion as a budding doc. After all, medicine is a field of service.

Remedying Imposter Syndrome

After accounting for all of the external and communal things that shape your development into a professional, there are some internal and individual growing pains that come along with your white coat too.

The biggest enemy in my first year of medical school was myself. Hands down. I was the poster child for imposter syndrome.

Imposter syndrome (IS) is the state of feeling like a fraud in a room of people who seem more competent than you are. It's a state of doubt that you are not supposed to be where you currently are, despite evident success. It is also a belief that you will eventually be found out or exposed when who you truly are doesn't add up to who you've "pretended" to be.

This can manifest as:

- Self-doubt
- Self- sabotaging
- An inability to properly self-assess competence
- An inability to accept or believe compliments
- Being overly critical of your performance
- Self-gaslighting (invalidating your thoughts, emotions, and behaviors)
- Attributing external factors, rather than personal qualities, to success
- Overachieving
- Experiencing anxiety when you do not meet realistic or highly-set expectations

Enduring waves of these "symptoms" is a normal part of medical school. When you think about it, everyone around you is just as smart and serious about their career as you are.

Requirements to constantly produce alongside other competent colleagues and classmates, external pressures, perfectionism, academic standards, ranking, competition, and social media are just a few things that may add to the pressure.

Plus it can be scary at times, and rightfully so, to imagine that you will be a full-fledged doctor, with *real* patients, in just a few short years.

You may be tempted to brush symptoms of IS under the rug to power through that test or clinical skills check. However, this feeling is a real thing; and, like in physical syndromes, tends to show up in multiple areas of your life.

Feeling like an imposter is NOT just "being hard on yourself" in the name of self-motivation, it is a form of self-sabotage that can quickly spiral and may stand in the way of you and your goals. I know this because I've been there, and still have these feelings from time to time.

Imposter syndrome can sometimes manifest as physical symptoms and mental health conditions such as depression and anxiety—which are reasons to seek professional help.

For the majority of first year, I was down BAD with IS, up to the very last day of classes. Some days were better than others, but there were many times when the feeling of being an imposter actually led me to believe that I wasn't good enough. If you feel this way too (even on the first day of classes) it is more common than anyone is willing to admit. But more importantly, it is possible to fight it and win.

Although these are in no way placeholders for professional help with IS, here are a few remedies that you can use to lessen the effects of it in first year:

Remedy #1 | Identify the standard you are trying to meet.
Identify the standard you are trying to meet. *Are you trying to get an 'A' on every test because that is how others define success? Is it because you are trying to keep up with your classmates? Is it because your parents— who may have no frame of reference for what you're going through— expect more*

from you? Who are you idolizing? Who are you performing for? How exactly are you not "adding up" in your head?

Remedy #2 | Refuse to be someone who doesn't exist.

Expectations can hurt the relationships you have with others and especially the one you have with yourself. Give yourself grace and recognize that any small victory — even doing your best despite the outcome–is worth celebrating in medical school. Contrary to popular belief, C=MD. *More of this on pg. 76*

Remedy #3 | Be inspired rather than influenced.

And yes, even by me. The worst thing you can do is try to copy and paste things into your life from the people you look up to. You are much more than a collection of others' ideas and advice.

Although it is great to have a pattern to follow, letting influence from others (standards, methods, appearance, etc.) overshadow your unique journey will leave you disconnected from who you are.

So a classmate or doctor did something you admire. Great! Let it inspire you to make it your own.

Don't conform to a mold that you were never meant to fit in.

Remedy #4 | Don't believe in what you see: deflect the impact of social media.

The success stories of med students and doctors on social media don't always accurately represent the waves of imposter syndrome everyone experiences during their career.

One reason for this is that genuine struggle isn't glamorous and doesn't always look good in a post, tweet, or TikTok. Also, the social standards put on doctors and med students to simply "be smart and successful" all of the time are reflected in social media, making it even harder to share the reality of what we go through on this journey.

When you think about it, social media is specifically designed to only highlight things that produce the "wow factor" for users (measured in likes and re-shares in favor of an algorithm). Even though social media may seem like a representation of reality, it isn't. That's why using it as a standard of comparison is so dangerous.

So again, realize that you are human and that you don't have to be as picture-perfect as the false examples you may consume on the socials. Comparison is the thief of joy.

Remedy #5 | Find community.
The strongest weapon against imposter syndrome is transparency. Instead of looking to the internet for answers, interact with real people. Find classmates and upperclassmen who are open to sharing their experiences with failure and how they've coped. Also, talk about your struggles (when necessary) to normalize them as a part of the learning process for yourself and others. You can also seek out interest groups and clubs to foster community around discussions about physicianhood that address the good AND the bad.

Layers of Self-Discovery

Who knew that the solution to being more successful in medical school has less to do with how much medical information you know and more to do with how much you know yourself?

As you can probably tell by now, the most important lessons you'll learn as a med student are life lessons.

First year may even kick off a season of self-discovery. This was my testimony because MS1 Ja'Neil did not know who she was. Truth is, not many people who start med school in their early 20s do.

For me, no amount of advice, good grades, publications, or awards made up for the lack of self-confidence I had when I started first year. I didn't see those outward signs of success compliment my journey healthily until I corrected internal patterns of negative self-talk, relearned who I was, and became comfortable with the reality of who I was becoming, This is another example of how self-esteem can influence the limits you place on your abilities. *What do you think about yourself? How do those self-generated or internalized messages affect how you navigate medical school?*

More than being bombarded and overloaded with advice and resources, knowing your triggers, limits, needs, and self-worth is the key to authentically defining the limits of your success. The hardest part of this process, however, is peeling back/evaluating all the layers that support (or don't support) your ability to learn and grow.

For example, the reason you got a question wrong on a quiz is not just because you didn't know the answer:

What kind of day did you have? What was sharing mental real estate with the concept you were trying to study? Did you shut down during class because you told yourself that the information was too hard? Are you unmotivated because you've become disconnected from the reason you applied to medical school in the first place? Are you too prideful to get help? Are you intimidated by the thought of being successful?

Let's be real, med school doesn't occur in a vacuum as much as people would like it to. More than you think, your capacity to learn has a lot to do with how you see yourself and how much you believe you can accomplish.

An extra layer: "Minority Mentality"
Most people can agree that believing self-generated non-truths is a problem, but internalizing stigmas reinforced by cultures, systems, and mass media can hold you back as a student and professional just as much, if not more.

I began my med school journey wondering if I would be able to perform at the same level as my classmates. On the surface, I knew that my qualifications and performance weren't limited by my race, gender, or my socio-economic status. But I couldn't help but feel pressure taking my first few tests knowing that based on the media and statistics, I— a twenty-two-year-old, black woman and child of two working-middle-class immigrants— was expected and primed to fail.

If I'm being honest, there were many moments when fulfilling my "minority stereotype" of being average, constantly struggling, and acting strong enough to do it on my own appeared to be the safest option. But chil', it was far from it.

Implicit biases that may exist within admissions committees aside, this is one example of how having a "minority mentality" can distort the idea of self. Subconsciously internalizing stigmas and stereotypes innate to systems and cultures can produce social anxiety, self-doubt, passivity, and or crippling pressure to prove the stereotypes wrong. This interplay between environment, behavior, and success is what experts call *stereotype threat*.[1]

This concept partially explains how someone can be socialized into believing that they can achieve more (or less) than is actually possible, or reasonable; and in turn, subconsciously alter their performance to make their belief true. *Crazy right?*

And no, not everyone is affected by this "threat", but it is something to keep in mind when understanding the origins of the internal limitations you might have. If this is affecting your learning experience/ professional development, please, I beg, find the support you need.

Despite these and other layers that may affect your journey, your job during first year is to know (or find out) who *you* are. Not who people say you are or who people expect you to be. Relearn yourself and let what you discover inform the kind of physician you want to be.

It's a marathon, not a sprint.

I know it may seem like I had it all figured out by the end of first year, but the truth is, I did NOT and I will always be on this journey of self-discovery— especially as it relates to how I will learn about and practice medicine. This is your formal invitation to join me there.

THE BOTTOM LINE(S)

What it means to "become a doctor" is an organic and nuanced process characterized by the balancing of personal identity with the current standard and accepted persona of a physician.

Learning how to effectively speak your truth as a med student can help you be a better advocate.

Many internal and external beliefs and behaviors can affect your professional growth. Identifying them is the first step to overcoming their effects.

Staying curious and involved will maximize your med school experience.

Additional Resources

1. Spencer, Steven J et al. "Stereotype Threat." *Annual review of psychology* vol. 67 (2016): 415-37.

Power Talk — Sarah Myers McGinty

Say What You Mean: A Mindful Approach to Nonviolent Communication — Oren Jay Sofer & Joseph Goldstein

Research Papers for Dummies

The Imposter Cure: Escape the Mind-Trap of Imposter Syndrome — Dr. Jessamy Hibberd

section 4
Creating a Balanced Med Student Lifestyle

There are so many moving parts of your life outside of med school that are necessary so you can function at your baseline. This year will be the first of many times you'll have to reinvent what "keeping it together" looks like for you.

Creating a Daily Routine

A daily routine is necessary. Since you will have to schedule your life around med school, start by picking one thing to do every day, then the rest of your day will fall into place (ideally).

I wish I had better news to tell you where this is concerned because my ENTIRE first year was trial and error to get my daily routine down to a science.

To create my routine, I started with a solid morning ritual that consisted of praying, devotion, personal hygiene, drinking tea, and mediation.

As I became consistent with that, I slowly extended the routine later on in the day until I had a full routine.

This changed many times to adapt to the COVID-19 restrictions that required me to attend classes in-person, then completely remote, and then via a hybrid style (in-person and virtual) by the end of the year.

Nevertheless, including at least one thing that grounded me every day was key.

Here are some things you can include in your routine:

- Morning playlist or podcast
- Spending time with God, or your higher power (see section on *Religion & Spirituality*)
- Tea/ Coffee
- Skincare routine
- Morning run or workout

When it comes to planning the rest of the day, or when you should go to sleep, know thyself:

- Stay consistent! Even your routine is one ritual
- Don't add too many things at once
- Include at least one thing that is restorative or brings you peace (e.g. a daily self-check-in or a five-minute power pose)

Caring for Your Crown

People don't typically acknowledge the amount of extra time that a sista (or a brotha) has to take out to take care of their hair during medical school, so I will— because it's an extreme sport.

Some weeks I showed up to class with my head wrap, sometimes with the wig, sometimes with a bun, and sometimes with that same bun but with a long braid pinned over it.

Whatever style worked, I did it.
(*Insert black girl magic meme here)

My biggest flex of medical school was conditioning my hair under my head wrap. It saved time instead of waiting for the deep conditioner to do its job, and rescued my sleep schedule so that my wash-day that turned into wash days was still effective .

Another unsolicited storytime:
I was so stressed out at the beginning of first year that my hair fell out. I wish I was joking, but I'm not. Thankfully, the headwraps doubled as a wash-day and "bald-J" hack that helped my scalp heal.

My hair routine was yet another thing I had to fit into my never-ending to-do list of first year. So, I committed to washing and treating my hair with natural pre-poos, serums, and treatments every week without fail. Thankfully, my hair grew back by the end of first year. I say all this to say that if your hair needs TLC to stay healthy, don't neglect it. Get creative and find different ways to keep your crown clean and moisturized.

Here are some ways you can fit hair maintenance into your busy med school schedule:

How to Create a Haircare Schedule

- Choose a **weekly** wash or moisture routine whether your hair is in a protective style or not (e.g. oiling/massaging your scalp)

- Choose a **bi-weekly** routine with more intense scalp or protein treatments

- Choose a **monthly** routine to give your hair a deep clean and moisture reset.

**Schedule these like you schedule study time.

- If you rock extensions, get creative with making the stages of protective styling work for you (e.g. if you have "old" box braids, refresh the front row or wrap them in braiding hair to turn them into faux locs)

How to Not Look Like Med School is Dragging You: A Systematic Approach to Outfits

Anyone who knows me knows that one thing I'm 'gon do is wear a full outfit to class. Every. Single. Time. It's just what I do and who I've always been.

Your school may require you to wear business casual attire to class (Don't panic I'll help you with that in a sec). Or, you may not be required to wear anything more than what you wore to bed. But as a student doctor, and professional-in-training, you need to start looking the part. Med school is your job. You never know what your day may bring and who you might cross paths with—a professor, a PI, or an attending who is looking for a mentee who's about their business.

Again, you don't have to buy super expensive things to meet that quota. You just need a few staple items, a steamer, and your sense of style.

Here are a few things you can try to maintain and upgrade your wardrobe during first year:

Balance versatility & comfort

Buy things that are super comfy and have clean lines and quality fabric. Doing so can make all the difference in the ease of putting together everyday outfits for multiple events. For example, slide-on sneakers can be paired with a casual outfit for on-campus study and can add dimension and comfort to a business casual outfit for class.

Color vs. Neutrals

Until recently, I have been afraid of color and patterns. I liked everything to match, so I would end up wearing some combination of browns and neutrals over and over again. There is nothing wrong with a neutral palette, but eventually, my closet ended up being the graveyard of all the colorful pieces I bought but never wore.
So I started small, started wearing colorful socks, resisted the urge to avoid patterns, stopped caring about "matching "and all of a sudden had more outfits to wear.

Have a theme

One thing that helped me continue this pattern, was having a theme in mind for the week.

Try hanging your favorite pieces and accent items in one section of your closet to visualize your options. Or randomly rearrange your closet when you get bored. Make it what I like to call, "the style lab".

Try capsule wardrobing

Once you choose a color scheme and a theme for the week, choose a few of your favorite items to create a capsule wardrobe and watch your looks come together:

How to Create a Weekly Capsule Wardrobe

- **4**-5 base items (your favorite jeans, or a white tee, a set of matching jewelry, or that jacket that seems to go with everything)

- **3** unique accents or "statement" pieces in your closet (a bright canvas bag, or a graphic tee with a message)

- **2** pairs of shoes (one comfy/ versatile pair, and one fancier pair)

- **1** layering item if needed (a light jacket or knit vest)

- **Pinterest:** If all of this sounds like too much, this message is for you: Pinterest boards save lives. When you're short on time and don't want to sacrifice style, download the app, make a Pinterest board and get some inspiration until outfit planning becomes effortless.

Re-purpose & up-cycle

I can't tell you the number of times I've made a dress into a top and tucked the rest into a high-waisted pant, or did the opposite and threw a tee over a jumpsuit to create a new look. This may be easier for women to do, but I've seen guys make it happen too.

Ain't nothin' wrong with a little thrift

Although you might feel a little strange wearing used items, finding good-quality, gently used pieces at a fraction of the original price is a great option if you want to refresh your look for the low. Before you thrift, go with a color scheme, a few looks, and a budget in mind.

Keeping Your Stomach (and Your Bank Account) Happy

In your first year, it's extremely important to save coins wherever you can. This means a food budget actually needs to be a thing. Believe it or not, it's twice as expensive and wasteful to try to make food at home while also buying takeout.

Now you may be thinking, how will I have time to make meals every day while balancing all the new material in first year? One option is a common solution: meal prep. Another is my personal favorite: have a handful of quick-and-easy recipes for each meal of the day that have a variety of substitutes. Whatever floats your boat will work, but it's worth it to try both:

Meal Prepping

Most schools don't have class on the weekends so this is a perfect time for you to make large portions of your favorite meals for the week ahead. Grab a deep saucepan and steam your veggies, season with fresh thyme and black pepper. Cut up your lettuce, peppers, and cucumbers so you can make quick salads for lunch. For meats, you can pre-season, section, and then prepare them fresh

in the oven or an air fryer.
I highly recommend investing in one because will cut your prep time in half and leave you enough time in the day to study.

Quick-and-easy meals with multiple substitutes

I started meal prepping but quickly got bored eating the same thing every day. So I chose meals with ingredients that I could easily switch out when I got bored.

- **Pancakes:** Complete pancake mix is my go-to for breakfast (because I don't eat eggs). To switch it up I toss some cinnamon and brown sugar on some days and chocolate chips on others. I pair it with a bowl of assorted fruit (which also varies from day to day). Some days when I get tired of the pancakes I pop the mix into a mini waffle maker.

- **Hot-pressed/ Stove-top paninis**: Another purchase that I will never regret is my panini press. My current go-to is sautéed mesquite turkey with Swiss cheese and sliced tomatoes on sourdough bread. You can't tell

me I didn't buy this from Panera. It's super easy to put together and takes 10 minutes total to make. No grill, no problem. A likkle butter in a pan will do the trick.

Alternatively, you can also add your choice of sauces to elevate the sandwich even more.

- **Rice:** You can pair rice with anything. Perfect that rice-to-water-ratio and pair with some fresh steamed veggies and seasoned chicken from your local market. Salmon with lemon is also a quick and easy meal that can be paired with rice and cooked in the oven while you watch a lecture.

- **Smoothies & spreads:** As you know, the options of fruits for smoothies and jams/ spreads are limitless. Blended smoothies and spreads (like fresh guacamole) are both great ways to sneak in fruits and veggies during the week in between the gallons of coffee and Red Bull.

Some of my other versatile meal faves were chicken salads for lunch and tacos for dinner.

Truth be told, there are some days when I was too lazy to make a meal, and all I end up eating is a bowl of fruit and a frozen pizza from Trader Joe's (heated up in the oven, of course). Striking a balance between take-out, meal prep, and fresh meals will pay off in the long run for your body and your pockets.

Pinterest, once again, has some quick, easy, and tasty ideas for meal solutions.

Also, remember to drink lots of water, exercise as much as you can, and take your daily vitamins!

Staying Connected to Your Higher Power: Religion & Spirituality

I get it, you may not be religious or spiritual; and the idea of squeezing church or mass into your med school schedule may be the furthest thing from your mind. This section is not in any way meant to convert you. This is simply my testimony of how I realized just how much I needed God in my first year; and how my faith in Him gave me the peace I needed to make it through in one piece.

When I got accepted into my current program, I wasn't exactly thrilled that I was going to a Christian school. After being in public school pretty much my whole life, I knew that the real world didn't revolve around religion, and thought that this Christian med school experience would deprive me of the traditional med student rights of passage. Plus, I had been raised in a Christian household and believed that a few prayers here and there were enough to help me pass my exams.

But I didn't realize that med school was a different beast and that surviving it would require me to rely on something greater than myself. You gotta remember my situation: new city, higher stakes, pandemic, no shortcuts. And I promised myself from day one that I was going to do this thing sober as a judge— no alcohol, no drugs, and no secret question banks.

The only sustainable option left for me was a personal and active relationship with God, Jesus, and the Holy Spirit; and I am convinced that this was the ONLY reason why I made it through all of the ups and downs of first year in my right mind.

It may seem like there is no time, and you may feel like your classmates have extra hours to study while you're at church or worship, but in reality, diligently setting aside time to be spiritually and mentally recharged will put you at an immeasurable advantage.

From sunset EVERY Friday night to sunset Saturday night (and sometimes until Sunday afternoon), I paused from ALL school work and school-related tasks. I wasn't behind and was just as successful (if not more) than those who plowed through the week without taking the time to reset and reconnect. If nothing I said struck a chord in you, lemme put it this way:

Whatever higher power brings you true peace, cling to it for dear life. Medical school is NOT the time to stop going to church. Or to stop praying. Or to stop observing your day of worship. PERIOD.

If you ascribe to religion or a spiritual belief in God, it is helpful to remain connected to those principles during medical school. This same faith will ground you when things get tough and doubts run high.

Ways to Stay Spiritually Connected

- Accept, believe, and bask in God's love for you. There is no use in relying on someone you don't believe in or have a relationship with.

- Have the prayer warriors you know on speed dial. Nothing hits different than a praying mama or auntie.

- Connect with a spiritual counselor at a nearby church

- Find a way to connect with God every day in the form of prayer or devotion

- Set a time to reconnect with God each week (e.g. church)

Here are a few Bible verses that have encouraged me thus far[1]:

- Matthew 6:25-33: Don't worry about what food you will eat or the clothes you need to cover your back... Look at the birds in the field. They do not plant or harvest but your Father feeds them. Don't you know that you are more valuable than they are?....

Seek the kingdom of God above all else, and all these other things you need will be given to you.

So don't worry about tomorrow. Each day has enough trouble of its own.

- **2 Corinthians 12:9**: His grace is sufficient and His power works best in weakness.

- **Romans 5:3-5**: We can rejoice when we run into problems and trials, for we know that they help us develop endurance. And endurance develops strength of character, and character strengthens confidence in a hope of salvation that will not lead to disappointment.

- **Philippians 1:6**: Be confident of this very thing that He who began a good work in you will carry it to completion until the day when Jesus returns.

- **Philippians 4:6-7**: Don't worry about anything, but pray about everything. Tell God what you need, and thank him for all that he has done. Then you will experience His peace that surpasses all understanding.

Making Sacrifices or Making Investments?

I can't count how many times I have been asked "how do you do it all" even before getting to medical school. Meanwhile, I can't tell you the last time I looked at my Twitter feed. I didn't even own a TV until months after first year. No matter how you slice it or dice it, being locked into medicine will require you to be out of touch with something for a while.

A cardiothoracic surgeon I shadowed years back told me, "You can have everything you want in this life, just not at the same time". Her words have stuck with me for years and have never failed to reset my focus.

I sacrificed things— some harder to give up than others— to avoid the regret of "if only I gave it my all" :

- Toxic relationships with "friends" and family members
- My (usual) hobbies, until my schedule was able to comfortably accommodate them
- Naps: Because of how my body is set up, I only took naps when I absolutely needed to.

- School activities/ positions: This may be a shocker to you, but I had to learn to say no to certain events, positions, and activities so I could get a few more hours of rest/ relaxation. *One thing I refused to sacrifice was sleep because if Ja'Neil is not relaxed, nothing productive is happening, okay?*

As much as I would like to sugarcoat the concept of sacrifice, some things will have to be removed from your life to protect your peace and to remain laser-focused on your goals during med school. Trust me, I tried to keep it all at first, and it took a toll on my mental health, physical health and most importantly, my edges.

In order to balance different things in your life as a med student, invest in a little wiggle room by making a few sacrifices. Make room for alone time, time to enjoy family, and enough time for a good night's rest.

What non-med-school-related things will you sacrifice to invest in your peace and focus?

Not Taking Yourself So Seriously

I am a perfectionist. I wanted to start medical school, something I've never done before, and miraculously do exceptionally well (don't we all). Some of my classmates appeared to succeed without breaking a sweat and that made me want to push harder than I physically could.

I knew in my heart that I was capable to do just as well, but what helped me do so was the COMPLETE OPPOSITE of what I thought would get me ahead. I thought I had to buckle down and make medicine my entire life. But really, sometimes I had to spend my last bit of energy on random dance sessions in my living room instead of studying. I had to schedule time for fun. I had to recognize and honor my humanness.

Make sure you laugh, make sure you cry, make sure you feel, make sure you're present, make sure you connect with those around you, and most of all, celebrate whenever you give your all, no matter the outcome. **Embrace your humanness, flaws and all, and give yourself grace.** Those are the keys to appreciating the beauty of this chapter.

Why Self-Care is King

In my first year, I became the queen of self-care. Every Saturday morning on my day off, I had on some type of face mask, put my phone on do-not-disturb, made myself pancakes, and put on my robe and essential oils. I set the vibe, watered my plants, spent time with Jesus, and pampered myself.

I made self-care a part of my routine and prioritized it right after eating and sleeping. I even made room in my budget for it. You should too!

You will fall apart in your first year, so it is extremely important to set aside time to relax and reset and care for yourself.

Try committing to one act of self-care (other than sleeping) each week of first year.

Being a Patient (If It's Necessary)

Mental and physical health is more important than being successful in med school. Being in optimal health is the best thing you can do to withstand the mental and physical rigor of class, tests, and training.

You can't be optimally productive if you are sick, tired, or both (true story). "Willing away" ADHD, depression, or anxiety doesn't work either. If you have dyslexia, social anxiety, or other conditions you've previously pushed to the side, now is the time to get support.

In the past, you may have been able to compensate. I get it. But I'm telling you, the stress of medical school *will* expose your weaknesses. In every way, shape, and form. It will push you to your limits. Med school is not for the weak (and by "weak" I mean suboptimal). I don't mean to scare you, but I'm keeping it real.

If you have any learning, physical, or mental conditions or disabilities, this is your sign to reach out and find the resources and support you need to function at your best.

It won't hurt to get a consult or take an inventory to get screened for common conditions that can hinder your learning experience.
I thought I was perfectly sane at the beginning of med school. But after taking a school inventory, I was humbled to find out that I had a ton of emotional issues I had never addressed: codependency issues,

depressive qualities, and anxiety.

This set off a warning bell that said "Hey sis, if you don't address your mental and physical health ASAP, you gon' crash and burn." If I hadn't listened or sought out the help I needed, I wouldn't have been in med school long enough to write this book.

Many schools like mine have an office for physician vitality or student counseling. If yours doesn't, they should at least have a directory you can look at to point you in the direction of help. *This is another sign to become familiar with what your insurance covers.*

Like I said in the context of learning earlier on, when it comes to maintaining your health, REACH OUT FOR HELP BEFORE IT'S TOO LATE.

Finding Your Tribe

The last piece to a balanced med student lifestyle is having a handful of people you can trust to give you support and objective advice and to be vulnerable with.
It may have worked in the past to

hear your mom say "it'll be okay, honey" to get you out of a season of self-doubt, but in this first year, however, your greatest support will come from those who are right there in the trenches with you.

Lean on a network of classmates and friends who will check in, guide you when needed, pray with you, be your sounding board, and be invested in your development into a successful physician and person.

The next two sections will dig deeper into how you can maintain these important personal and professional relationships.

THE BOTTOM LINE(S)

It is possible to live a sane, balanced med-student lifestyle.

You are in complete control of your priorities during medical school. This means if you want to get eight hours of sleep, you will get it if that is important to or necessary for YOU. One of my mentors said it best: **Triage your life.**

Daily routines are the anchor for habits that complement your life as a student.

Be consistent with meals, your self-care routines, outfit choices, worship time, or methods of self-reflection. This will give you the grounding that you can fall back on when school becomes overwhelming.

The goal should be to not have ANYTHING in your life that you don't absolutely need (relationships, habits, negative self-talk).

Don't front on God if you know Him to be your most reliable source of strength.

Many of the lifestyle sacrifices you'll have to make in med school are actually investments.

Working on being a whole person will help you be a better student and doctor.

If you aren't honest about who you are or what you need, you may forfeit the necessary support to become your healed and authentic self.

Know when to lean on your support team. You don't have to be or feel alone.

In reality, there may be things out of your control that may prevent you from finding moments to take time for yourself or to reconnect to your humanity; but don't let that be your excuse not to try. You only fail when you give up. Simply put, if you want to do this doctor thing while maintaining a balanced lifestyle, *you got's to see it through my boy.*

Additional Resources

1. Holy Bible: International Children's Bible. Dallas, Tex: World Pub, 1988. Accessed with *Bible* App for iPhone.

Good Mornings: Morning Rituals for Wellness, Peace and Purpose — Linnea Dunne

Fast and Easy Five-Ingredient Recipes: A Cookbook for Busy People — Philia Kelnhofer

Medical Student Well-Being: An Essential Guide— Dana Zappetti & Jonathan D. Avery

The More of Less — Joshua Becker

The Power of Full Engagement— Jim Loehr & Tony Schwartz

Mamba Mentality: How I Play— Kobe Bryant

section 5

Maintaining Your Circle in Med School: Setting Boundaries in Your Personal Relationships

Boundary setting is another thing that may seem like a pointless task in the grand scheme of first year, but is a big step you'll have to take to get your priorities in order.

Boundary Basics

Learning how to set boundaries is the heaviest, yet most valuable lesson to learn in the first year of med school (and any other professional program for that matter). For me, it was tough to do so because first-year me was so afraid to take up space; I had never done this in such a drastic way before.

Before med school, I had always fit into people's expectations in relationships. I was the golden child, the friend you could always count on, a great listener, etc. And because a good number of people in my life benefit from this, I didn't have much experience setting healthy boundaries.

At the very beginning of school, it was easy to continue checking in and being involved in every family matter and staying up late keke-ing with my girlfriends.

But eventually, I became conflicted with making enough time for myself and my career while also spending time to maintain the relationships that sustained me to get to where I currently was.

After a boatload of self-talk, therapy, and prayer, I decided to set clear boundaries to balance my relationships with people *and* my relationship with my calling.

I had to have hard conversations. I had to learn to say no. I had to learn to not apologize for putting my phone on do not disturb. I had to ignore some calls and texts completely.

Cutting people off is not the solution

Now, this boundary-setting thing is not just for people you want to keep out of your life, but more so for those who you want to keep in it.

No one wants to tell their mom that they can't make it home for the annual family event. No one wants to keep rescheduling time to catch up with a friend. The reality is though, school won't let up from here on out, so it's up to you to choose between setting boundaries, or constantly being torn between your commitments to school and loved ones.

Is it uncomfortable? Yea. But is it necessary? Absolutely.

Boundary setting is an intentional feat, one that requires some thought, empathy, and communication. It is walking a fine line between giving as much as you can to develop your career while also nurturing vital relationships with people who helped you get to this point.

The best advice I can give to you when setting boundaries with anyone is:

- Know your limits.
- Act like they exist.

Triage your life like you will triage your future patients

(Had to throw in a few nods to my mentors who are amazing emergency medicine docs.)

Triage is the assignment of degrees of urgency to wounds or illnesses to decide the order of treatment of a large number of patients or casualties.

In other words, everyone is sick, but some are sicker.

Circling back to why this metaphor fits the concept of boundary setting: the relationships you triage higher aren't more important, but are more relevant in this stage of your life.

Setting Boundaries with The Fam

You may be great at triaging already which is awesome, but it is an ongoing process that I know can be hard or even awkward to do with the fam—especially if they may not fully understand what this journey entails.

This means that you probably shouldn't update them on your grades if you can't handle the extra pressure. Or if you KNOW you won't get much-needed study time at home you probably shouldn't go home for Thanksgiving break.

After evaluating what is necessary for you to function at your best, communicate this to your family.

Lovingly educate them, communicate what you need, and don't feel bad for making room for you. From now on, you're always going to feel like someone needs something from you, but you can't pour into others if your cup is empty.

The parentals

The hardest part is the tension that will arise when your parents have to relearn the person you're becoming.

As frustrating as it may be for you to have parents who might not understand the lifestyle changes you've made to adapt to med student life, it is just as uncomfortable for them to see the same person who once needed them to change their diaper operate as a fully-functioning adult and have peoples' lives in their hands.

However awkward and comfortable this process is, it is necessary to maintain relationships with your parents, siblings, and loved ones.

Be patient. Try your best to not get frustrated with your parents if they don't know what med school is like. A few months ago, you didn't either.

Even before medical school, explaining to your loved ones how you expect your life to change and all of the feelings that come with that process —anxiety, fears, and concerns— may help your family better accept the boundaries you set.

Setting Boundaries with Friends: "The Shift"

The fact that your friend group is getting smaller is NOT a sign that you're a bad friend. It just means that you are growing up.

At the beginning of every major life event (marriage, a new child, starting med school) is a shifting of your closest and not-so-close friendships. Sometimes for the better, and sometimes, not so much.

It may be worth your while to take an inventory of which friends bring meaning to your life during first year. Not the friends from undergrad who became your friend just because it was convenient, not the friend who just hits you up to party or when they need something, and definitely not the one who always finds a way to pull you into unideal situations.

Keep the "day 1". The for-lifer, the ride or die, & the low-maintenance friend. The ones who push you. The people who align with the core of who you are. Mentally relabel all the others as your acquaintances and treat them as such. Don't waste the energy on friendships that are one-sided, draining, or ambiguous.

In other words, prioritize, maintain, and grow your true friendships.

Although this seems extreme, you have every right to be selective because your career is at stake.

Your real friends will understand that this season in your life requires the highest possible level of focus. And hopefully, they match your grind within their own life and can easily relate to your need to set boundaries in the first place.

In my first year, it didn't take long for me to realize that I needed my real friends to remain sane. Shutting them out was never a solid option, and wasn't even a thought in my mind when figuring out what and who I would have to sacrifice.

Again, I had to be honest about how much time I would have for my friends in this new chapter and prioritized the ones that added value to my life.

As for the friends who I grew apart from; they are still in my prayers and my heart, but in a different way. They were given a lower triage tier in my life, and that's okay.
Hate to say it, but don't hate to see it.

For your circle of friends who survive the shift during the first year, set a recurring time to talk to them. Love on them. Affirm them and the relationship. Be present when it's time to talk or spend quality time. If they are a true priority and the feeling is mutual, be intentional about keeping them in your life.

Setting Boundaries with Your Significant Other

I cannot give much wisdom in this department because I was not in a romantic relationship during my first year. But many of my classmates were out here wifed-up or boo'd-up with whole relationships, in-laws, and even kids.

The one thing I do know is that the first year, the "easiest" year, sets the foundation for how your relationship will grow as your list of responsibilities gets longer. For those who begin first year in a committed relationship, don't you worry, I've talked to some people who were in your shoes. Below is the gist of what they've taught me:

- **Know thyself:** For example, if you know you are easily distracted, or spend more time complaining about how hard med school is when your boo is around, communicate this to them and find ways to get in some solo study time.

- **Intentionally date your partner:** When setting dates: it's **quality over quantity**. Plan to do things with your partner that strengthen your relationship (check-ins, bonding activities, sit-down dates, couples therapy sessions, etc.)

- **Set clear expectations and commitments:** This applies to you whether you are in a committed relationship or not. If you want to date just to go out and look cute, say that. If you want something more, say that too. Being unclear about your intentions will cause you a lot of heartache and confusion that you can't afford.

If you are in a relationship, let your partner know how much quality time they can expect from you. Let them know what commitments you are willing to make, or what type of support you may need them to be. Also, be open to compromise.

- **Take them on the journey with you:** Explain your goals, how you plan to achieve them, and most importantly, how they fit in the grand scheme of it all.

- **Be okay with knowing the right person at the wrong time**: If you are dating (because I am not suggesting you do this if you're married or have kids) recognize that sometimes the right person—no matter how fione he or she may be— may come into your at a time when you need to be in grind mode. Sometimes you can't compromise or communicate it out. Sometimes your schedules clash too much.

The plain and honest truth is that some relationships won't survive this chapter, and shouldn't be revived if they are incompatible with your life as a medical student. *If there was an amen corner for that, I would be all in, up, and through it.*

Singleness is not a dirty word, especially in med school

Cues Living Single title sequence
Periods of singleness are valuable stages that will allow you to discover yourself, so you're as whole as you can be when you start a new relationship. That means, if you are single, DO NOT search for a relationship just because you are bored or lonely after you get done with studying. That's toxic energy.

Singleness is also a time to evaluate the pros and cons of dating medical and non-medical students and to learn from those who are just as successful in maintaining relationships as they are in their careers. Singleness is not an "in-between" sentence to purgatory but is necessary to have healthy romantic relationships period.

Setting Boundaries with Yourself

The relationship you have and the boundaries you make with yourself are just as important as the ones you have with loved ones. When you set self-boundaries—how much time you take to decompress, how much grace you give yourself, how much negative self-talk you allow

or positive self-talk you require,
etc.—it teaches the people in your
life how to honor them. It will also set
the standard for the new personal
and professional relationships you
cultivate during and after medical
school.

Setting these kinds of boundaries is
another form of self-care.
This means that you'll have to
make the word "no" a part of your
vocab. And yea, I know we've already
covered this in the last sub-section,
but this piece of advice is important
enough to say again.
Make room for you.

THE BOTTOM LINE

It is possible to maintain and even deepen the friendships and meaningful connections in your life during first year.

Triage your relationships like you will with your future patients. Doing this may require you to make hard choices and sacrifices about who and what to give your "free" time to.

Setting boundaries with others is a form of setting boundaries with yourself. Protect ya peace at all costs.

Additional Resources

Off Balance—Matthew Kenny

Boundaries: When to Say Yes, How to Say No to Take Control of Your Life— Henry Cloud

Life Matters: Creating a Dynamic Work Life Balance of Work, Family, Life, and Money— A. Roger Merrill and Rebecca Merill

Love in the Time of Medical School: Build a happy, healthy relationship with a medical student — Sarah Epstein

section 6
Student-Doctah Networking &
The Power of Bonding Upwards

While building relationships with your family and classmates is important, connecting with upper-level students, residents, and attendings is just as essential.

If you look hard enough, you'll find people who've successfully navigated the places you hope to be in. Connecting with them will put you in the best position to gain the wisdom and motivation you need to build a career.

With time, the upperclassmen and physicians I connected with during my first year went from being great resources and mentors to amazing friends. They put me on game, helped me explore my new community, and shared valuable experiences that put both my academic and personal goals in perspective.

The Ten

The summer before starting medical school, I read *The Memo: What Women of Color Need To Know To Secure A Seat At The Table* by Minda Harts. In the chapter "Building Your Squad", she talked about the "Top 8"—a solid handful of business or professional contacts everyone should have to call on for advice, counsel, or expertise.

Auntie Minda was onto something. This concept is one that I highly recommend you adopt as you begin your medical career interacting with a bunch of experienced and connected doctors and professors every day.

My med school version of the "Top 8" is **The Ten —a group of 10 colleagues, physicians, and professors who you can rely on to give you moral, academic, or financial support throughout your med school journey.**

You're a professional now and professionals are supposed to know other professionals. Also, a major part of this med school journey is building a one-of-a-kind career around your degree. A great way to start is by connecting with people who can give you the constructive criticism you need, encourage you to push your limits and dream bigger, pull strings in high places, and support your goals along the way.

"The Ten" is fluid, and may change as you grow into your career. Here are my current ten:

- Best friend, 4th year pharmacy student (P4)
- Friend, MS4
- Friend, 1st year resident, cardiology

- Mentor, OB-GYN attending of 20+ yrs, department chair
- Mentor, emergency med attending & residency director
- Mentor, cardiologist attending, sextuple board-certified (I don't have to list them all, but you get the point)
- Mentor, physician-scientist, and artist
- Family friend, Executive VP of a hospital system
- Family friend/ father-figure, federal judge
- Family friend/father-figure, Doctor of Education

Everyone in my "ten" is in their BAG, okay? I am blessed beyond words to have these amazing professionals in my corner.

The goal is to know a variety of professionals you can call up, bounce ideas off of, and chat with. Ideally, your ten will become the innermost circle of your professional network.

After you identify your ten, check in with them from time to time. Let them know how you're doing. Maintain and leverage those relationships.

Online Networking is a Must

COVID-19 has made online networking a necessity in pretty much every professional field. Everyone is on social media, and new features make it easier than ever to build your brand to network on social media platforms.

Updating Your Profiles

Make sure your social media profiles are updated. Here are a few ways to upgrade your digital reputation and brand yourself as a medical student:

Update your headshot

Make sure to have a solid, head-on, non-selfie headshot—this is very possible especially with how good smartphone cameras are these days. With some good natural lighting and a pressed shirt, aim to have a headshot that screams "I'm going to be somebody's doctor one day".

Update your Curriculum Vitae (CV)

(FYI, a CV is a complete record of your credentials, while a resumes is focused for a specific position.)

- Get rid of anything from more than four years ago that is not relevant to your career or that you did not continue
- Get rid of any side-hustles (like the time you did hair or sold t-shirts off the books) in the employment or "professional experience section" unrelated to your professional skill-set
- Include and emphasize all research projects and presentations

Update your current social media profiles

- Make sure your @ name is easy to find (avoid extra characters)
- Consider creating a professional account or getting rid of any social media content that doesn't reflect the professional you are becoming
- When posting and reposting content, be clear about the movements and causes you support and do not support (silence also speaks loud)
- If you want to post you partying, drinking, or whatever else you do, make a finsta (a fake, private Instagram account followed by friends who won't snitch to admin). Don't risk getting in trouble with your school for violating anything that may be in your student contract unless

you are willing to deal with the consequences.

Get familiar with workflow apps that will help you stay connected

- GroupMe
- Slack
- Monday
- Smart Sheet
- ClickUp

Step up ya email game

- Update all of your email signatures with your contact info and med student status
- Use your school email for all professional/ school-related email threads
- Learn how to construct clear emails (you can ask one of your "ten" for feedback to help with this)

Get active on apps that can help you strengthen your online network

- LinkedIn
- Clubhouse
- Facebook Groups
- Fishbowl

Also, PLEASE figure out how to navigate Zoom, Microsoft Teams, and Google Meet. It doesn't look like the need for online video meetings is going anywhere, so try your best to get comfortable with the various tools and features for each platform before you use them (so it doesn't get in the way of your meetings and presentations).

Shoot your shot

If there is a group or person you would like to work with or learn from, don't be afraid to hit them up via a direct message or email. You'd be surprised how many doors can open as a med student (shadowing, research, and leadership opportunities, student committees, or partnerships, etc.) from interactions on social media.

How Your Social Media Presence Can Count In Med School

Recall that when I talked about imposter syndrome earlier on, I mentioned social media and how comparing your journey with what you see on those platforms is a possible source of discouragement.

However, taking advantage of the positives of social media by having a prominent (heavy on the prominent) presence or platform is now a way to measure your impact during medical school. If you have found a way to impact the world of medicine through tweets, posts, YouTube videos, or blogs, do it, and do it well. Residencies are beginning to acknowledge the value of having social media influence. This new trend in medical education is a real thing and is called "Digital Scholarship". Look it up, and thank me later.

Professional Relationships with Professors, Advisors, & Mentors

It may be scary and even foreign to rub shoulders with the folk in charge. But, just remember you are your best advocate.

Now I'm NOT suggesting that you kiss anyone's butt. What I am saying is put ya big boy pants on and get to know the people who will hand you your degree in four years.

While there is always a group of students who just seem to be very connected, focus on your journey. Also, know that there is no reason why you can't be connected too, if you want to be.

Here are examples of a few people you might want to get to know in your first year:

Faculty
Knowing at least one faculty member from your med school's admin is important because:
- You can get more accurate information (about grading policies and whatnot) than by word of mouth from classmates
- They will know your name and vouch for you
- Recommendations for honor societies and residency will be easier to get if you have relationships with the professors and administrators who've watched you grow. Also, great letters of recommendation are LIKE GOLD because many tests and curriculums have switched to a pass/fail grading system.
- You will feel more empowered to create relationships with other admin that may become part of your circle (or even your 10)

Advisors
Keeping a good relationship with your department advisor can give you tailor-made feedback about your professional and academic performance.

Once you get to know your advisor, use the time you have with them to discuss your academic goals and to create/tweak game plans to set them in play.

If you don't leave their office feeling empowered, humbled (because good advisors will tell it like it is), or feeling like you can conquer the world, find a new advisor. Period. You don't have time to waste being without the academic support you need.

Mentors

Find a professor/doctor or two on your assigned rotations or electives in a specialty you're interested in and spark a conversation. Start by asking them what it's like to be in their shoes or what it takes to get where they are today. Or you can straight up ask them to be your mentor.

Doctors (with real-life patients and busy lives) rarely ask med students to be their mentees, so put yourself out there (maybe in one of the settings we talked about in section 3) and find yourself a mentor or two who will tell you what it's like to do their job every day.

Also, don't underestimate the value of having mentors in science-adjacent and non-scientific fields. These relationships can build your knowledge and reputation in multiple professional spheres.

THE BOTTOM LINE

Your grades won't get you as far as they used to— but a solid network will.

Additional Resources

How To Work A Room: The Ultimate Guide to Making Lasting Connections—in Person and Online—Susan Roane

The Memo: What Women of Color Need To Know To Secure A Seat At The Table—Minda Harts

section 7
Staying Where the Money Resides: Financing Med School

You either:

A. Kept rockin' with me throughout all of my rants and random stories and you've finally made it to the last chapter. Thanks for being a real one.

B. Skipped around to this section because getting your coins together in med school is a high priority. I respect the hustle.

Either way, the key takeaway from this section is short and sweet:

Money should be your LAST concern during medical school.

"But how? I didn't get a scholarship"
"But how? My mom told me that no debt is good debt"
"But how? I can't work while I'm in school"

Aht aht. Before you start finding reasons why my statement seems impossible, I have one more story that will hopefully give you the confidence to set yourself up for financial stability during and after medical school.

Disclaimer: This is in no way shade thrown at my school, BUT the workshop we received about spending and borrowing money instilled the fear of God in me. That day, the presenter said a lot but all I heard was "DON'T SPEND MONEY or else the $10 pizza you buy today will be worth $10,000 in loans by the time you start residency".

That is not financial literacy, it is financial fear. (Again, no shade)

You'll probably be required to attend these seemingly pointless and fear-provoking sessions too. Don't get me wrong, these will provide you with some gems, but take the advice given during these sessions with a grain of salt.

I, tragically, did not.

For about a week or two after the session, I budgeted HEAVY. I calculated how much interest would accumulate on EVERYTHING I bought down to quick trips to the coffee shop and snacks before spending. I started to withhold things I enjoyed from myself because I was afraid that I would somehow blow through my whole loan disbursement in a month.

Sad, right?

I did that at first because until then, I had never borrowed so much money in my life (and I just knew my Jamaican ancestors were rolling over in their graves as soon as I hit "accept" to borrow so much instead of getting a job). Also, in my mind, the word "budget" was supposed to be something necessary but equally uncomfortable. As a result, I suffered in the first few months and missed out on the comfort that a good budget was supposed to give me. Looking back, I'm diagnosing my past self with "spending cyclothymia": characterized by the back-and-forth of feeling guilty for spending too much when you aren't and not feeling guilty enough when you go over budget. Sounds familiar?

Eventually, I realized that there was no way to live like that for the whole year, had a reality check, and restructured my budget.

I'm not even 'gon front, even after finding a balanced way to follow my budget, I did not become an expert at managing my coins all of a sudden. Why? Because I was working toward my medical degree and was not getting my degree in finance.

I kept up with a realistic budget, but things still came up. My car battery randomly died, I flew home at the last minute for spring break, and my apartment's AC unit decided to act up and drove my electricity bill up to a crazy high one month. It turns out that the real key to budgeting is being able to appropriately adjust it when life happens. So when trying to get your money together, making a simple plan that can adjust to the twists and turns of real life is more than enough to stay in the black.

In other words, beloved, if you want to buy that pizza with loan money, buy it. Live your best life. Buy two even, but next month, make sure to make up for it by cooking an extra meal or two at home.

A Crash Course on Loans

A major contributor to the back and forth of my spending habits was the misunderstanding of how loans work and how I could use them to my advantage. Some other factors included the obvious guilt and fear instilled in me by my upbringing and not being shown what a healthy relationship with borrowed money or credit looks like. But it was time to be an adult and make my own decisions, which sucked.

Yes, it is great to have mom and dad on speed dial in case you're short a hundo for this month's rent, but med school is the best time to learn how to manage a budget with the amount of money/credit in your name or account. The first step is becoming friends (not enemies) with your loans.

These broke-med-student principles helped me overcome the ill feelings I had against the money I borrowed:

Broke-Med Student Proverbs

- Loans aren't just debt, they are investments.
- A budget is a safety net, not a jail cell.
- Sometimes needs will be expensive, and it's okay if it can be made it up in the next months.
- What is borrowed out is all that should be spent (Calling the parentals for help should be the LAST resort)
- Credit cards are a flex if used properly (e.g. points/cashback)
- And again, for good measure, money should be the last concern. There are so many other things to worry about.

I don't come from a lot of money or trust funds and all of that, but leaning on those principles resolved a lot of my budgeting problems within a matter of a few months.

If the things on that list didn't comfort you enough, here are ways to set up a solid budget in first year.

1. Set a deadline to total your money

When planning out your finances, it is very important to set a deadline for yourself (based on the posting of all of your school scholarships, grants, graduation money, etc.) to get a definite total of how much money you'll be working with for the first year.

And I'm not talking about the money your uncle Joe said he was going to give you, nor the money you might get from the scholarship you applied to over the summer. You should just consider the money you ACTUALLY have by the date you set for yourself.

2. Determine your needs

To start outlining your budget, start by listing your absolute needs, NOT wants. Here is a standard list that can give you a place to begin:

Housing
- Rent
- Electricity bill
- Gas bill
- Water
- Trash
- Internet/cable

Other Necessities
- Food
- Groceries
- Dining out (SUPER IMPORTANT SO YOU DON'T GET CAUGHT UP)

"Credit-Killers"
- Car note
- Car insurance
- Phone bill
- Credit card bills

In a normal budget, a savings category would be included, but if you can save money while taking out loans, you should return the extra money you have. Remember, the extra money you "save" is accumulating interest from the moment it hits your account.

3. Give yourself a (structured) cushion for your wants

The part at which people usually play themselves is when they (and when I say they, I also mean me) do not budget "fun money" for little trips to the mall, snacks, and skincare products. Those dollars and cents really add up.

If you don't trust yourself to do this, there are a bunch of financing apps that can provide you with more tangible accountability.

Also, using a credit card for these purchases can give you structure, and will light a fire under you to be more conscious of your spending habits.

4. Apply for fee assistance
Although you are no longer eligible for a Pell Grant (loans you don't have to return) as a grad student, the FAFSA still has to be filled out for you to receive your loans **every year** you are enrolled. Apply for your FAFSA as soon as you can (always due by 6/30).

FOOD STAMPS: After you get over the stigma of "government cheese", apply for food stamps. This can save you a lot on groceries. You may be eligible if your loans are your only "source of income". (Also, the stamps now come in a discrete debit card form.)

5. Consider your borrowing options
I will also assume that you, like me, didn't understand all that went into borrowing money for school or where to find all of this information. In the heat of applying to get all of the long lists of things for registration out of the way, you may have missed the important parts of the loan entrance counseling. Don't worry, I'll break it down for ya:

Interest Rate: Percent of the loan that will be incurred (accumulated or added to your overall loan) for borrowing the actual money itself.

APR: the amount of money that it will cost you per year to borrow the money.

Sounds like the same thing as the rate right? The APR is the actual dollar amount that includes any additional service or processing fees.

Total Cost of Attendance (COA): This will determine the upper limit of what you can borrow. Loan money IS NOT UNLIMITED and is determined by this amount. This is the estimated cost of tuition and fees plus the cost of living expenses based on your school and the federal requirements they have to follow.

There is more info on this at studentaid.gov

Now that you have a plan and know all of the fancy terms, here are a few options that you have when borrowing (from lowest interest rate to the highest interest rate):

Your Money: the best interest-free option, if you can afford it.

Direct Unsubsidized Stafford Loan: This was offered to you in undergrad too, but this time you won't need to show proof of your financial need to qualify for this loan. This type of loan has the lowest interest rate. You can only borrow up to the COA amount determined by your school. The interest on the money you borrow will collect the moment the money hits your account.

GRAD PLUS Loans: Also lent to you by the federal government and capped by the COA determined by your school; these will fill in any additional financial gaps not covered by scholarships, grants, or unsubsidized loans.

Private Student Loans Through A Credit Union or Bank: Credit-based loans with crazy high interest rates. Please DO NOT borrow money for school this way unless you absolutely need to. This is a last-resort option. (Better yet, just avoid this option at all costs.)

Scholarships

Some websites and funds offer scholarships and grants to medical students. Although they are far and few, they are out there and can help you reduce the loans you take out each semester.

Also, remember the admin you're supposed to know in the dean's office? Ask them about any extra grants and scholarships they may have too.

Med Student Scholarship Tips

- Keep a few of your personal statement drafts close by to save time when writing scholarship essays.
- Apply for 2-3 med school and non-med school scholarships every month. Don't be too proud to apply for those "small" awards
- Apply for a mixture of merit-based and essay-based scholarships
- Search for specialty-specific scholarships: there is so much money given every year to med students who are committed to certain specialties (awards for the folk who want to go into primary care and family medicine are easiest to find).

- The National Medical Fellowships Scholarships & Awards Program automatically finds medical scholarships that fit your profile.
- Consider service scholarships: The National Health Service Corps Scholarship Program is also an option that will cover tuition, fees, and living expenses if you agree to complete a few years of service in an underrepresented community following/ during med school. If you've already taken out loans and are still interested, NHSCP also offers loan forgiveness if you meet specific criteria
- Again, stay in the loop with your dean's office so that you know when new scholarship opportunities become available.

The Truth about Working Part-Time Jobs

Medical school is a full-time job. Being as Caribbean as I am, I considered finding an extra job in addition to school to help with my bills. It also didn't help that for the first few months my family kept asking when I would find an extra side hustle.

I'm sure it can be done (and shout out to my classmates who did) but if you don't absolutely have to, **don't take on a part-time job. The money you'll make will never be worth more than the bit of sanity you'll have left from being a med student.**

Your free time is extremely limited and you should be dedicated to mental and physical rest. I'm begging you, at least until you get through first year, don't bite off more than you can chew.

THE BOTTOM LINE
If you are smart about your borrowing and spending habits, it WILL be worth it to take out loans in medical school (if you can't afford to pay for it in cash)

Borrow exactly what you need because you will have so many other things to stress out about in first year.

HIGHLY RECOMMENDED RESOURCE
The White Coat Investor's Guide For Students: How Medical and Dental Students Can Secure Their Financial Future—James M. Dahle

Your Last "Real" Summer

Before you know it, your first year will zoom by. Summertime will roll around again and you'll be one giant step closer to achieving a goal that has been years in the making. The beautiful thing is that if you attend a med school that gives you a summer "break" before second year, the summer is a time to do literally whatever you want.

You can use this last summer to do research, shadow, complete a preceptorship, or volunteer. OR you can be *outside* like I was (when I wasn't slaving over this book): going to day-party-after-day-party, exploring new cities, and going on random day adventures and road trips.

This is the last "real" break you'll get before second year (which is a beast), so choose wisely and PLEASE GET SOME REST. Whatever you do make sure you do something meaningful and restorative—even if your thing is sleeping.

Farewell, Future Doc

If you made it this far to the end, I'm hoping that you got all of the advice you need to kill first year. If you don't remember anything from this guide, remember that it's a marathon, not a sprint, and that more than any strategy you learn or use, remaining connected to who you are and why you started this journey is the secret sauce. Trust me, it all will be worth it the day those two extra letters at the end of your name grant you the ability to positively impact patients, their families, and their communities. I'm rooting for you.
Keep pushing and don't give up.

Until next time *wink wink*,

—JGMH

P.S. Before you go, as promised, there are a few sections following this page that might be helpful throughout the year.

FIRST YEAR CHECKLIST

Here is a checklist of things you should handle before you start your first year:

- ☐ See your primary care physician (PCP) to get:
  - ☐ A physical
  - ☐ Required vaccinations for your specific school
  - ☐ A copy of your vaccination record (for your files)

- ☐ See any other specialists for check-ups (e.g. dental cleanings or the gyno for the ladies)

- ☐ Check your health insurance coverage to make sure that you will have access to the same benefits in the city where your school is located

- ☐ Complete all school registration items before the registration deadline to avoid extra fees:
  - ☐ Free Application for Federal Student Aid (FAFSA)
  - ☐ Your school's financial aid application and forms
  - ☐ Submission of tax forms to your school (if required)
  - ☐ Loan entrance counseling on the Federal Student Aid website
  - ☐ Sign your Master Promissory Note (also on Federal Student Aid website)

- ☐ View your school's policy on car registration (you may have to re-register your car in the state you'll go to school in)

- ☐ Register your car with your school's parking service

- ☐ Get familiar with your student portal (e.g. Canvas, D2L). It's helpful to get your log-in for the portal saved and notifications turned on, especially for the first couple of weeks

- ☐ Write all of your most important ID numbers, passwords, and codes in a safe place

- ☐ Temporarily change your mailing address or forward your mail to your apartment or dorm

- ☐ Update your driver's license and other forms of ID (e.g. passports)

- ☐ Get a copy of all of your important documents:
    - ☐ Vaccination record
    - ☐ Passport
    - ☐ Insurance Cards

- ☐ Set a monthly budget *(see section 7)*

- ☐ Square away any debt from credit cards or past-due bills

- ☐ Check your credit score and credit report for any suspicious activity

- ☐ Save all of the following numbers on your phone:

    - ☐ Dean's Office
    - ☐ Student Health Services
    - ☐ Financial Aid / Student Accounts
    - ☐ Counseling/Student Supp
    - ☐ Campus Security
    - ☐ IT Services

- ☐ Complete any state or federal training for compliance, confidentiality, or work conduct required by your school

- ☐ Clear space on your phone, laptop, and other devices
    It may be helpful to organize all of your documents and have your important files (digital receipts and signed forms) and information (CV, resume, headshot, bio) all in a folder that's easy to get to

☐ Get the supplies you *actually* need (*see section 1*)

☐ Update your social media profiles (*see section 6*)

Anything else?

I probably missed a lot of other things that you will need, but the least I can do though, is give you space to write them down. Here you go:

☐

☐

☐

☐

☐

☐

☐

☐

☐

Med Speak Glossary

The words and phrases used by med students and doctors can be confusing. Some of these terms don't make any sense at all but are helpful for you to know (so you don't just nod "yes" when you don't have a clue what a doctor is saying to you). You're welcome in advance. *Other terms were defined in text (e.g. PI, LO)*

Doctah-ing it up: pronounced "dahk-tuh-ing it up" (heavy on the doc, soft on the "-or"); the act of blending one's authentic self with the persona of a physician

Code-switching: changing the way you speak, act, or interact with others depending on the context (workplace, school, formal events, etc.); a survival tactic used by minoritized individuals to be accepted in predominantly white companies and institutions

Gunner: that student who is doing THE MOST to be at the top of the class no matter what; a student who is always trying to outshine the rest by answering questions first or dominating conversations to impress your superiors. Gunners often lack social cues. You'll always hear an earful about how disappointed they are to receive anything lower than 90% on tests as if that is not good enough. They usually undervalue the concepts of teamwork and mediocrity (Don't be a gunner; it's not always worth it)

Zebra: A common phrase is, "When you hear hoofbeats, think horses, not zebras,". Because we med students are taught so many rare conditions, it is easy to quickly misdiagnose with the rare conditions (the zebra's) first. Consider more common diagnoses (the horses) before the rare ones.

Streak: Anki term for how many days straight you've completed all of your reviews

High-Yield: describes the information that is super important for you to know or is likely to be on boards

MOA: mechanism of action; describes the way a drug acts in terms of the cellular components or biochemical pathways it targets

Pass/ Passes: Some people use this term to describe the number of times that they have reviewed information or lecture content (e.g. "I gave embryology three passes this week").

Short coat: the white coat that first and second-years get before they start their clinical rotations (*not standard across all medical schools*)

Long coat: the white coat that third-years and beyond wear to denote their clinical training (*not standard across all medical schools*)

Didactics: usually referring to your pre-clinical years: the first year or two of med school during which learning is achieved via lectures and assessment tests

Formatives: All med students are evaluated are via summative assessments— tests and grades; you may also be evaluated via formative assessments — learning inventories and benchmark assessments that evaluate your learning process and understanding of topics.

Clerkship: practice-based learning mode for third and fourth-years; a name to collectively describe the required rotations that happen after didactic learning

PDx: Physical Diagnosis lab; where you'll use physical maneuvers (e.g. using your stethoscope) to help you diagnose conditions. The skills you learn here will help you prepare for your OSCEs.

OSCE: Objective Structured Clinical Examination; how you will be tested on the skills you learn from PDX against the national standard

Differential Diagnosis: abbreviated ddx; a list of conditions a patient likely has based on the physical exam and or interview findings gathered by a clinician

SOAP note: Subjective, Objective, Assessment and Plan; an official document of written communication between health care providers about a patient; these won't always be fun to write but are necessary to correctly document a patient's case; most widely-used method of charting.

SBAR: Situation-Background-Assessment-Recommendation; a shorthand way of effectively communicating between health care providers about a patient's condition

HPI: History of Present Illness; the information that should be obtained from a well-conducted patient intake interview. You'll learn how to properly retrieve this in your physical diagnosis (PDx) / clinical skills lab; this is included as a part of the SOAP note

"Presenting" a patient aka "Chiefing": The act of giving a short summary or report of a patient —using the relevant/ important info you gain from the HPI and patient interview— to your superiors (residents, attendings, etc.). This can often be intimidating but will get better with practice.

Pimp, v.: stands for "Put in my place"; a questionable term to describe when attendings or residents put med students on the spot (usually in front of peers) to test their knowledge about a specific condition. When it's your turn to be "pimped", be confident. If you rise to the occasion, they'll be impressed, if not, well, good luck next time.

Rounds: a time when the residents present the status and updates on their patients, discuss treatment plans and interventions, order and stop meds, visit, and check up on patients, all under the attending's supervision; usually happens in the morning with the attending and residents.

MDR: Multi-Disciplinary Rounds. Some services may conduct MDRs with PAs, social workers, nutritionists, PTs, etc. depending on the relevance of their immediate input to patient management.

In-patient: requiring a patient to be admitted into the hospital; fun fact: the emergency department is not considered to be an in-patient service

Out-patient: outside of the hospital; not requiring a patient to be admitted into the hospital; e.g. free clinic

Service: another word for department or unit (e.g. "I'm shadowing on the surgery service today")

Rotation/wards: time spent working on a specific unit or service; rotations specifically referring to your third or fourth-year clinical experiences but can also be used to describe any assigned time on a service

Scut: scut work is busywork no one wants to do, but is still vital to the management of patients; tasks that seem "below your pay grade". Until you're an attending (see hierarchy below), you're likely to be "on scut" if that is what you're told or required to do.

HIPAA: no, this is not the animal that looks similar to a rhino; the Health Insurance Portability and Accountability Act of 1996 is a federal law that protects patient information and has strict guidelines on who has access to Protected Health Information (PHI); the reason you can't take photos or videos in the hospital (unless you're not showing any patient information). Your school will definitely have some training on what is considered PHI and how to make sure you are not violating these very strict laws.

OSH: outside hospital; a hospital not within the hospital campus you are in

BIBA: brought in by ambulance

ED: emergency department; same thing as emergency room; emergency docs prefer ED because there are more rooms in one in the department (might be obvi but this is their preference)

OR: operating room

PI: principal investigator: This person is in charge of research labs. They may be clinical MD doctors or PhD doctors or both. Reach out to them or their office when you are interested in being a part of a research project they're leading.

IRB: Institutional Review Board; an institution's FDA-approved committee of experts and administrators who regulate biomedical research involving human subjects; they are the governing body over all research projects (and funding) done at each academic research site

NIH: National Institutes of Health; the country's medical research agency; an organization that funds and conducts the largest research projects in the nation

Pubs: short for publications; research submitted to peer-reviewed research journals

Step: referring to one of three (previously four) USMLE (United States Medical Licensing Exam) step-wise board exams that you will need to take throughout your training (Step 1, after year 2; Step 2- after year 3; Step 3-during PGY-1). Students usually take Step 1 after or during their last didactic year (traditionally year 2). Step 1 is based on basic science knowledge (all of the facts you crammed to learn) and the later board exams will cover more clinical-based material as you rotate through each department in your clinical years (usually years 3 & 4).

Shelf Exam: specific subject examinations after third or fourth year rotations offered by the NBME (for MD students) and NBOME (for DO students)

NBME: National Board of Medical Examiners (or Osteopathic Medical examiners for NBOME); the organization that evaluates allopathic medical students and residents through the USMLE exam and Shelf Exams; basically the folk who write and regulate step and shelf exams

ERAS: Electronic Residency Application Service; how 4th years apply for residency

FREIDA: AMA's Residency and Fellowship Data Base; has all important information about residency programs; you have to pay for FREIDA, but there are a few free ones out there too (e.g.. *residencyexplorer.org* via AAMC)

Match Day: This is the day that every med student looks forward to. This is the day that fourth years get matched through an algorithm based on their rankings to a residency program in the specialty of their choice.

All of the ICUs (may also be pronounced "ik-YEW" if followed by a letter representing a specific type of ICU; e.g.. PICU is pronounced "pic-YEW"): Intensive care units with critically ill patients who are usually on life-support, machines, heavy medications, or are under strict monitoring

"Steezh": a nick-name for Anesthesia

ROAD specialties: an acronym for the most competitive specialties: Radiology; Ophthalmology or Orthopedic Surgery, Anesthesia, & Dermatology

PPE: Personal Protective Equipment; required masks, caps, and gear used in the in-patient setting for certain floors or departments.

WHO: World Health Organization; they are an agency of the United Nations that oversees matters of international public health. They also regulate the standardized practices and regulations of medical sub-fields (e.g. classifications of tumors, operating room time-out protocols)

You should also familiarize yourself with common medical abbreviations and terms not only used by med students or doctors but all types of health care professionals; especially if you are rotating on in-patient units
(e.g. npo= nothing by mouth or bid= twice a day)

The Hierarchy of Medicine

Here is a breakdown of the medical food chain from "bottom" to "top"*:

Pre-med: Someone who is currently completing requirements to apply to medical school; this is not a major, but is a track.

MS or M (insert number 1-4): Represents the year of medical school a student is in:

> **M1 / M2:** Pre-clinical student. They mostly learn via lectures/exams.

> **M3 / M4:** Clinical student; most of their learning happens on the floor (in clinical settings) rather than from a textbook; they are on required rotations for the majority of the year

Sub-Intern: A fourth-year med student on their sub-internship (abbreviated "sub-I") —a clinical rotation at which fourth-years are heavily evaluated; basically an audition for residency which may or may not be at the hospital associated with their med school

Resident: A doctor who has completed medical school but is currently training in a specific specialty or subset of medicine. They are paid (although not that much) to train under an attending. They rotate on services depending on their specialty; designated by PGY (insert number) year. PGY stands for "post-graduate year". *Back in the day, residents used to live in hospitals (hence the name)*

Intern: First-year resident; they start in July and rotate on other services that are related to their specialty.

Charge Nurse: They are the leader of the unit on their shift and know the ins and outs of the department; they handle discharges and transfers of nursing staff; they are also the point person in the OR (so make sure you introduce yourself to them in addition to the docs when you shadow, esp. in the OR)

Chief resident: the requirements and appointment of this title depends on the specialty; usually a senior resident who is appointed (based on performance) who is in charge of the interns and has more administrative responsibilities; when the attending isn't there, they are in charge

Physician's Assistant (PA): No, this is not someone who opted to be an assistant because they couldn't get into or finish medical school. The PA track is a separate and equally important field. What sets PAs apart from physicians is that they have to complete a six year Master's program, take a different licensing exam (PANCE), and have to be supervised by a physician to make clinical decisions.

Attending: They are the big kahuna. The boss. They have completed residency, and are typically the lead doctor on a patient's healthcare team. They supervise, train, and teach a group of residents.

Fellow: An attending who is undergoing additional training in another residency program.

Board-certified physician: The GOAT. The expert. They have gone above and beyond to surpass the minimal requirements of training in a specific specialty. Their passing score on an oral or written exam, which varies between specialties, ensures that their medical practice and knowledge were approved by a college (or group) of other highly-regarded docs.

*This list does not intend to cover all valuable team members and clinicians on a patient's healthcare team.